W

Fit

and

Sexy

for

Life

The Hormone-Free Plan for Staying Slim, Strong, and
Fabulous in Your Forties, Fifties, and Beyond

Fit
and
Sexy
for
Life

. . . .

Kathy Kaehler

with Stacy Whitman

Broadway Books   New York

W

The instructions and advice in this book are not intended to take the place of medical advice from a trained medical professional. Readers are advised to consult a physician or other qualified health professional regarding treatment of their medical problems and before beginning any exercise regimen. The author, publisher, and recipe writer disclaim any liability or loss, personal or otherwise, resulting from any treatment, action, or application of a medicine, herb, or preparation to any person reading or following the information in this book.

PUBLISHED BY BROADWAY BOOKS

Copyright © 2007 by Kathy Kaehler

All Rights Reserved

Published in the United States by Broadway Books, an imprint of The Doubleday Broadway Publishing Group, a division of Random House, Inc., New York. www.broadwaybooks.com

BROADWAY BOOKS and its logo, a letter B bisected on the diagonal, are trademarks of Random House, Inc.

Book design by rlf design
Photographs by Erik Asla

Library of Congress Cataloging-in-Publication Data
Kaehler, Kathy.
    Fit and sexy for life : the hormone-free plan for staying slim, strong, and fabulous in your forties, fifties, and beyond / Kathy Kaehler. — 1st ed.
        p.   cm.
    1. Exercise.   2. Physical fitness.   3. Health.   I. Title.
RA781.K23   2007
613.7'1—dc22
                                                           2006022440

ISBN 978-0-7679-1618-9

PRINTED IN THE UNITED STATES OF AMERICA

10 9 8 7 6 5 4 3 2 1

First Edition

To my sisterhood connections

May the relationships, stories, and experiences

that you've shared with me resonate in each one of us

and thread us together as stronger and

more powerful women.

Contents

Fit
and
Sexy
for
Life

Introduction

A s s o m e of my best female friends and clients have confided, it seems to happen overnight: Suddenly, one day, you feel like a different person. You're snapping at your kids one minute, and breaking down in tears the next. You feel sad and angry and cranky and tired, and you can't explain why. All you know is that you don't feel well—and looking in the mirror makes you feel even worse. Your skin looks dry and wrinkled, and you can barely button your pants. To top it off, you've been waking up in the middle of the night drenched in sweat. Is it really any wonder that you haven't had a decent night's sleep in weeks?

Welcome to the midlife roller-coaster ride known as menopause. Yes, *menopause*. Because in this book, you won't hear me refer to it as "the M word" or "the change." Whether you're just starting to skip periods or you haven't menstruated in months, it's time to face and hopefully even embrace this inevitable right of passage. From now on, let's stop pretending that it isn't happening, refusing to talk about it, and dealing with it alone. Because it happens to all of us—and there are a lot of things that we can do to ease the transition.

Unfortunately, the hormonal and physical changes associated with getting older can take a real physical and emotional toll. As your body starts producing less of the female hormones estrogen and progesterone, your risk of heart disease, breast cancer, and osteoporosis increases. And as you no doubt already know, you can be plagued by side effects ranging from weight gain (especially around your middle) and achy joints to hot flashes, sleeplessness, irritability, and painful intercourse.

But trust me: It doesn't have to be that way. With the right diet and exercise program—one geared specifically toward your body's changing needs—you can control your weight; boost your energy; and protect your heart, bones, and breasts through your forties, fifties, and beyond. What's more, you can manage those irritating menopausal symptoms, including hot flashes, fatigue, and mood swings, so they don't wreak havoc on your life. As you'll discover on the following pages, all it takes is a few simple *(really!)* lifestyle changes to start feeling strong, fit, and balanced again.

For decades millions of women have used hormone therapy (HT) to ease hot flashes and other side effects. But new studies have questioned the widespread use of HT. The bottom line: While hormones may work for some women, they aren't right for everyone. That's why I've developed a natural alternative for coping with unpleasant symptoms and keeping us young and healthy.

The New Aging: Fit, Fun, and Sexy!

Thinking back to my childhood, I vaguely remember my mother referring to menopause as "the change." "I'm going through 'the change,' " she would say. I had no idea what she meant. Was she going to change into something other than my mom? And then there was "the flash." What was that? Suddenly, she would get hot and start fanning herself, pulling at the collar of her shirt and seeming exasperated.

At age forty-four, I have yet to experience a hot flash. But I have started to notice my periods getting lighter and more erratic. In my twenties and thirties, the blood would start flowing on the twenty-eighth day of my cycle, like clockwork. This past month, it arrived on the fifty-ninth day! *Could I be pregnant?* I asked myself. Maybe, but most likely not. It must be perimenopause, I concluded. My period is going away. My period that I have loved and hated. My period that has shaped me as a woman. My period that gave me the ability to have my three children.

Over the years, I've found that women rarely talk about their periods in a positive way. As a young girl, I can recall being really scared about menstruating for the first time. I didn't want to be the first one to get my period, but I didn't want to be the last, either. I also remember some of my friends referring to it as "the curse." But menstruation is a powerful part of our life journey. It carves and sculpts our way into womanhood. In a sense, our menstrual cycles are our calendars, our way of tracking time. It's something that we anticipate every month, and it can dictate our mood, our appearance, our weight, and whether we're pregnant.

As my own childbearing years come to a close, I'm surprised to find myself feeling sad and strangely lonely. I never knew that I would feel this way. How can the absence of my periods make me feel so different? Does every woman feel like this? Am I crazy? Or are the emotions that I'm having normal? I wonder if these are the same questions that my mother posed to herself a few decades ago.

At the same time, I feel so incredibly lucky to have such a sensitive and supportive partner—my husband of thirteen years and the love of my life, Billy Koch. I also have three beautiful sons—my ten-year-old twins, Cooper and Payton, and my six-year-old, Walker. Sometimes it's hard for me to accept that I won't be having another child. I'll never change another diaper, never see my belly grow again. To think that I won't get to live that experience again makes my heart ache.

But with that said, I'm absolutely determined not to let these changes get the best of me. Yes, I'll allow myself to grieve the loss of my fertility. But I won't look at this as the beginning of the end. And I refuse to start slowing down. Instead, I plan to leap into the next chapter of my life with energy and gusto. I'm going to continue exercising almost every day so I feel great and love my shape. I'm going to up my intake of calcium and be sure to get the other nutrients I need to stay strong and healthy. I'm also going to have fabulous sex *and* be the one to initiate it. In other words, I won't be pausing for menopause—and neither should you!

My Fit and Sexy for Life Plan

I've been healthy and active all of my life. But in the last few years, even I've found it difficult to fit exercise into my schedule. Between my career and family life, there just isn't much time left for me. With my one-on-one personal training business, regular fitness segments on NBC's *Today* show, a bimonthly newspaper column, a company called Health-E-tips, and a fitness class that I teach four times a week, I have about five jobs. I also have four dogs and three kids, so I know a little something about stress and scheduling conflicts.

I've also been gaining weight in places that I never gained it, and finding those excess pounds harder to lose. Part of the reason is that my metabolism is slowing down. Because this is such a busy time in my life, I've become less attentive to my fitness program. But this is no time to start letting it slide; after all, I know better than anyone that exercise is essential to minimize my waistline, as well as many of the other side effects of aging that may be on the horizon.

Believe me, I'm familiar with the monthly hormonal fluctuations that can make you want to break down in tears in the middle of Target or crawl into bed in the middle of the day. If it weren't for daily exercise to de-stress, I'd be a complete wreck—and no doubt, my work and family life would suffer. That's why all of my books, this one included, highlight easy ways to sneak physical activity into your life. In my experience, if it's hard to fit in, no one will do it.

That's where my Fit and Sexy plan comes in. Designed specifically for perimenopausal and menopausal women, my program combines walking and strength training to eliminate unwanted pounds, rev up your metabolism, and cut your risk of heart disease, osteoporosis, and other conditions. The exercises are easy on your joints and are designed to boost your mood and energy level, rather than wear you down. After all, we need energy to get through our hectic days, because the pressures of life, work, and motherhood certainly don't stop when our periods do.

As our bones become brittle with advancing age, falling is a real threat that can result in broken bones and fractures, a long healing process, and a brutal rehabilitation program. This is why my workout plan includes lots of squats and lunges to build strength and improve balance. These exercises come in handy if, let's say, you're standing on the curb waiting for the Walk sign, and you fall off. These balance-boosting moves will help you catch yourself without spraining your ankle or breaking a hip.

When I set out to write this book, I experimented with different exercises. Then I put them together like pieces of a jigsaw puzzle to see which ones fit and how they flowed. I wanted the moves to address some of the classic problems of women in our stage of life, from flabby arms and wide buttocks to love handles where slender waists once were. My Fit and Sexy plan pays special attention to the abdominal region, which tends to expand during menopause. I'll give you the moves to tighten and tone your midsection, and teach you how to really zero in on your target muscles for fast results.

I've also included exercises to strengthen and tone your pelvic floor. You can do these daily—say, when you are driving to work. These exercises, called Kegels, can make sex more enjoyable and, as you get older, lower the risk of embarrassing accidents that can occur when the pelvic floor muscles that support your bladder are weak.

Being all too familiar with time crunches, I knew that the program had to be simple. Face it, we don't have hours to spend working out, and we don't always have the ability or the desire to go to a gym. So you'll find that while the moves themselves may not be new, the way that they work with your lifestyle is. There aren't any complicated routines or fancy equipment. They are just easy but effective exercises that you can do either at the gym or in the privacy of your living room.

I've done all of these moves with dozens of women—including celebrity clients such as Michelle Pfeiffer, Julia Roberts, Cindy Crawford, and most recently, Kim Basinger—and have seen amazing results, especially when Fit and Sexy is coupled with a low-fat, high-fiber eating plan. The changes to your diet are supereasy to incorporate; I know because it's the same way that I eat every day.

As you read on, you'll learn that there are ways to manage just about every aging symptom that nature dishes out, from hot flashes to bone loss. Beginning with small changes and working up to a whole new you, Fit and Sexy will give you the tools to look as young as you feel, and feel as young as you look. And I'll show you how to do both as seamlessly as possible.

In researching this book, I've learned valuable lessons from some of the wonderful and wise women in my life—including my own mom. In the pages to come, I'll reveal their thoughts and advice on this monumental life passage. By telling their stories—and opening up about my own experiences—I hope to help you feel better about the changes that your body is going through, and understand that you aren't helpless. This may be a crazy time in our lives, but we can control it. Over the hill? All dried up? Past our prime? Forget it! Together, let's prove that these years *can* be fun. No matter what your age, you can be fit! And you can be sexy!

1
. . . .

Your Changing Body

A Head-to-Toe Guide

ONE THING that I have learned about getting older is that every woman's experience is unique. For some, it can come with a tremendous sense of freedom—freedom from menstrual periods, childrearing responsibilities, and worries about unintended pregnancy. For others, it can be filled with feelings of sadness, anxiety, shame, and loss—the loss of our fertility, our femininity, our figures, and our looks.

Likewise, there's a lot of variability when it comes to the physical and emotional side effects. Approximately 75 percent of women report some troublesome symptoms, but the type and severity can vary drastically from one to the next. For example, some women are plagued by night sweats and insomnia, while others never have a single hot flash or lose a wink of sleep. Some start noticing a change in their periods as early as their thirties, while others continue having regular menstrual cycles until they're well into their fifties.

I have to admit that before I started working on this book, menopause was a bit of a mystery to me. I really didn't know what to expect, or how it might affect me, and that was just fine. I vaguely remember my mom going through it, though I didn't realize the significance at the time. And of course, when you're younger, it's the furthest thing from your mind. But now that I'm on the brink of perimenopause myself, I realize that it's important to understand what's happening to my body. After all, knowledge is the key to staying healthy and getting through the changes that lie ahead.

Demystifying Menopause

Literally speaking, menopause is the time in your life when you stop having menstrual periods. *Meno* comes from the Latin word meaning "lasting a month"; *pause* comes from the Greek word with the same meaning. In other words, a pause in monthly events. But it really isn't an event that occurs suddenly, without any warning, as the definition implies. Rather, for most women, it's a change that happens gradually over a period of years.

The first stage of menopause, known as *perimenopause,* is when the changes and symptoms typically start. During this time, your ovaries begin producing less *estrogen* and *progesterone*—hormones that play important roles in ovulation and menstruation. Estrogen causes the *endometrium* (the lining of the uterus) to start to thicken in preparation for a fertilized egg. Progesterone prepares the lining of the uterus for the implantation of a fertilized egg. If a fertilized egg does not reach the uterus, the endometrium is shed as a menstrual period.

As their estrogen and progesterone levels drop, most women notice their menstrual cycles becoming irregular. You may skip a period, or experience lighter, heavier, shorter, or longer flows than usual. This shift in hormones also affects other organs and systems in your body. The result can be disturbing side effects including hot flashes, headaches, mood swings, and forgetfulness. It also may cause problems such as achy joints, urinary incontinence, and vaginal dryness.

Menopause Glossary

Premenopause—the reproductive years following puberty.

Perimenopause—the transitional stage spanning roughly two to ten years before menstruation ends. Even if your periods are irregular, you can still get pregnant during this time, though it is less likely than in your twenties or thirties.

Menopause—once twelve months have passed since your last period, you've reached menopause.

Postmenopause—the years following menopause.

Induced menopause—menopause that occurs as a result of surgery to remove the ovaries or certain drugs and treatments such as chemo-therapy or radiation.

Early or premature menopause—natural menopause that happens before the age of forty.

Throughout perimenopause—which can start as early as your thirties and last up to ten years or more—your levels of estrogen and proges-terone continue to decline until your menstrual cycle stops for good. Once twelve months have passed since your last period, you've reached menopause. On average, this stage occurs between ages fifty and fifty-one, but it can also happen much sooner or later. You're likely to go through menopause around the same time that your mother, grand-mother, or sister did, give or take a few years.

In the final stage of menopause, which is called *postmenopause*, those hot flashes and other menopausal symptoms usually begin to ease up. But unfortunately, now that your body is producing less estrogen, your risk of heart disease, osteoporosis, and breast cancer is higher—which is why it's more important than ever to take care of yourself and make any necessary lifestyle changes to stave off these deadly diseases.

For most women, menopause is a natural biological process that occurs with age. But it also can be caused by surgery to remove the ovaries and certain medications and treatments, such as radiation and chemotherapy. These are typical reasons for menopause in women under age forty. Low levels of estrogen and damage to the ovaries can also cause early menopause.

In previous centuries, few women lived beyond menopause. But today, with a life expectancy of 79.7 years, we experience at least one-third of our lives after menopause. By 2020, the number of American women older than age fifty-five is estimated to be 45.9 million, compared with 31.2 million in 2000. As our life span improves, so does the

Seeing Red?

While you may expect your period to get shorter and lighter during perimenopause, many women experience an increase in bleeding. So don't be surprised if your menstrual cycles suddenly become longer or heavier than normal. According to the North American Menopause Society, this can be a perfectly normal occurrence. However, abnormal bleeding also can signal another problem, such as an ectopic pregnancy, thyroid disease, uterine fibroids or polyps, endometriosis, or cancer. You should be sure to check with your gynecologist immediately if any of the following occurs:

- Bleeding is very heavy, especially with clots.
- Bleeding lasts longer than seven days, or two to three (or more) days longer than usual.
- You have fewer than twenty-one days between periods.
- You have spotting or bleeding between periods.
- You bleed after sex.

accepted wisdom about menopause. Rather than being the beginning of the end, I like to think of menopause as the end of the beginning.

But Wait, Aren't I Too Young for This?

A few years ago, when my good friend Carolyn, a forty-one-year-old real estate broker, didn't get her period, she started to panic. Her menstrual cycles had been regular since puberty. She'd never skipped a period except at age twenty-four, when she was pregnant with her twins. You could set your clock by her menstrual cycles, she often joked.

It occurred to her that she could be pregnant, but she quickly banished the thought from her head. Not only are she and her husband careful when it comes to birth control, she'd just finished reading an article on how difficult it is for women to get pregnant after age thirty-five. Then she had another intrusive thought. What if she had cancer?

She quickly dialed her gynecologist's number. He didn't seem concerned. "It sounds like you're showing the signs of perimenopause," he told her. Carolyn was stunned. She was approaching *menopause?* She told herself that it couldn't be possible. She was in great physical shape, training for her second marathon. At work and at home, she felt sharper and more energetic than ever. It was that simple. She was too young for menopause.

Carolyn remembered all too clearly how weepy her own mother was when she went through menopause. She would have a hot flash at the dinner table and then lie on the kitchen floor to cool off. Her mother often felt faint and dizzy and complained about it for years. Carolyn didn't feel anything like that. Not even close.

Carolyn's doctor suggested that she start keeping track of her periods in a diary or on a calendar. He also asked her to note if her flow was heavy or light or lasted longer than usual. He asked her to come in so he could run some routine tests. That's when he took a complete history and ran blood tests to rule out other conditions such as pregnancy and thyroid disorder.

He also did a blood test that measured levels of FSH (follicle-stimulating hormone). Produced by the pituitary gland in the brain, FSH helps regulate the growth and development of our eggs and follicles. However, in menopause, those eggs and follicles don't develop. So the pituitary gland releases more FSH, hoping to push the ovaries into action. This is why a high FSH level may be the first clue that you're approaching menopause.

Sound simple enough? Well, there *is* a catch. During perimenopause, your FSH levels can fluctuate wildly as your estrogen levels wax and wane—from month to month and even from day to day. So your doctor may need to do more than one FSH test to attain useful information. Even then, the results may be misleading. The bottom line: The only way to know for certain that you've reached menopause is if you've gone twelve consecutive months without having a period.

If, like Carolyn and me, you've been noticing changes in your menstrual cycle, or experiencing symptoms such as insomnia or hot flashes, I recommend scheduling an appointment with your ob-gyn or primary-care doctor. Keeping a diary to track changes in your menstrual pattern is also a good idea, so you can see when and where changes occur and share them with your health provider. I've been doing this ever since I was in college on the advice of my gynecologist. To this day, I record the start date of each period in my Filofax. You might also want to write down how many days it lasts and whether it's light or heavy.

Keep in mind that not all bleeding irregularities are caused by perimenopause. As noted earlier, abnormal menstrual cycles can be a sign of thyroid disease, uterine fibroids or polyps, or even cervical or uterine cancer. To pinpoint the exact problem, your doctor will probably order a blood test to check your FSH level and thyroid. You may also be advised to get a Pap smear, a transvaginal ultrasound, or an endometrial biopsy, depending on your symptoms.

If your physician suspects perimenopause, however, he or she may order certain screening tests, including ones to measure your cholesterol level and bone density. If you're experiencing any unpleasant or unusual side effects—no matter how embarrassing they seem—you'll want to mention them and ask about possible treatments. Be sure your doctor

Six Questions to Ask Your Doctor

Women's health expert Donnica Moore, MD, of the nationally syndicated radio show *Dr. Donnica's Women's Health Report* and president of DrDonnica.com, a women's Internet health resource, recommends asking your doctor these questions when you hit perimenopause:

- When can I stop worrying about birth control?

- Do I need to make any changes or adjustments to the medication that I currently take?

- Given my personal and familial risk factors, for what conditions do I have an increased risk? (Osteoporosis, heart disease, cancer, and Alzheimer's disease are just some of the conditions you may want to discuss.)

- What screening tests will I need and when?

- What signs and symptoms should I be watching for?

- Is it safe to begin an exercise program or continue my current program?

Many women are confused, shocked, or in denial when they realize that they're approaching or in menopause, and may not remember to ask these important questions. Jot them down on a piece of paper or an index card before you visit your doctor. Write down the answers so you can refer to them in the future.

knows your medical history—including whether you or any of your immediate family members have had heart disease, osteoporosis, or breast cancer.

Managing Your Menopot

I'm a very active person, and always have been. Because I exercise so much, I rarely have trouble maintaining my weight. That is, until recently. Now that I'm in my forties, my body is changing. Even though I'm eating the same amount that I used to, my pants are getting tighter, my hips are getting wider, and I'm gaining weight around my middle. Recently, I even popped the snap on my favorite jeans.

Sadly, I suspect I'm a victim of middle-age spread. And I'm certainly not the only one. According to some estimates, the average woman gains ten to fifteen pounds during her menopausal years. Most of this comes on slowly, about a pound a year after age thirty-five. Wait—we're supposed to be gaining wisdom with age, not weight!

. . . .

"Menopause takes one into the territory that can be a victory for the bigger Self. But the Ego can pay a huge price."

—Molly, age fifty-three

. . . .

For years, some experts believed that hormones were to blame for the added pounds. But new research suggests that our sedentary lifestyles and overeating are the real culprits. As we get older, many of us start becoming less active. Consequently, we lose muscle, which causes our metabolisms to slow—so our bodies burn fewer calories. Over time, this can add up to extra inches, especially if we don't curb our eating habits.

In one study, researchers examined the weight of 485 women ranging in age from forty-two to fifty. They found that the women gained an average of about five pounds over a three-year period. The weight gain occurred regardless of whether the women were going through menopause—an indication that declining estrogen levels weren't a major factor.

Hormonal changes can, however, affect where our excess body fat is stored. As estrogen levels drop and we begin producing more of the hormones androgen and testosterone, the storage site of fat shifts to our abdomen. In her book *Fight Fat after Forty*, Pamela Peeke, MD, MPH, former senior scientist at the National Institutes of Health, refers to this phenomenon as a "menopot." Even if you've had a flat belly all of your life, you may suddenly find your waistline expanding.

I don't know about you, but I'm not ready for a menopot! The good news is, we have the power to do something about it. By exercising and eating right, we can stave off those excess pounds, as well as shed the weight that we've already gained. My Fit and Sexy for Life program combines walking and strength training to burn fat and build muscle, which is the key to a supercharged metabolism. I've also included special abdominal exercises to firm and flatten your belly and keep the menopot at bay.

Is Anybody Else Hot in Here?

My childhood friend Marie, now the owner of a small gift and novelty store in a Pennsylvania suburb, got her first taste of menopause in the form of a heat wave—and not the tropical kind. She just got hot, for no apparent reason.

Ever since Marie was a teenager, her periods were irregular, so she didn't notice any changes in her cycle at first. The hot flashes, however, caught her attention. She'd be watching television or doing inventory at her store, when out of the blue, she'd break into a sweat. The first time it happened, she was ringing up a picture frame for a customer. Suddenly her face turned bright red, and she began sweating so much that the hair around her face was soaked. She had no idea what was happening. Neither did her customer. The kind woman asked Marie if she should call 911 or bring her some water. The flash lasted for about three minutes. Marie was so embarrassed that she didn't charge the woman for the frame.

As time went on, her flashes became more frequent—sometimes occurring three or four times a day. Marie had to give up coffee and tea because they seemed to trigger her flashes. She also said good-bye to spicy foods. As much as she loved curry and chimichangas, they proved to be catalysts for her flashes.

Hot flashes like the ones that Marie describes affect as many as 85 percent of all perimenopausal and menopausal women. They can last anywhere from a few seconds to several minutes, and can occur multiple times throughout the day. They're characterized by a sudden feeling of warmth or intense heat, mostly on your head, neck, and chest. While their cause isn't completely understood, they're believed to be the result of a sudden change in your hypothalamus—the part of your brain that regulates temperature—which is brought on by the loss of estrogen. When your hypothalamus mistakenly thinks that your body is overheating, it starts a chain of events to cool you down: your heart beats faster, your blood vessels dilate, and your sweat glands start pumping.

Hot flashes can be mild: a feeling of warmth that comes over you, then quickly disappears. Or they can be intense: your heart starts racing, your face turns bright red, and perspiration starts pouring down your face. Flashes can be preceded or accompanied by a racing pulse, dizziness, anxiety, headache, or nausea. They can seem to come out of nowhere, or they can be triggered by stress or things such as spicy food, red wine, and coffee—just as Marie discovered. They can happen at any time of day, but they're most likely to strike in the morning and evening.

Hot flashes can also hit during the wee hours of the night. In a survey by the National Sleep Foundation, more than a third of menopausal and postmenopausal women reported suffering night sweats as they slept. On average, the hot flashes occurred three days per week and interfered with sleep five days per month, according to the survey of 1,102 women, ages thirty to sixty. When they disturb your sleep, night sweats can make you even more tired, irritable, and downright hard to be around.

Hot flashes tend to be more intense among women who have had induced menopause (through surgical removal of their ovaries or ovary damage caused by certain drugs or radiation), as well as women who have an early natural menopause (before age forty). Women who are obese are less likely to develop hot flashes, because some estrogen is available from their fat stores. Very thin women tend to fare worse. (But don't think this is an excuse to hit the cookie jar!)

Hormone therapy (combined estrogen-progestin or estrogen only) is still considered the most effective way to treat severe hot flashes. In fact, research shows that it can reduce hot flashes by up to 90 percent. But there are also other tactics—including exercise and avoiding triggers such as coffee—that can help.

Anatomy of a Hot Flash

Whether you've experienced the sudden wave of what seems like a thousand degrees of heat or just heard tales of woe from your friends and colleagues, this quick primer on the hot flash will help you understand how it can affect your body.

1. Your hypothalamus, a gland in your brain that controls body temperature, reacts to dips in your blood level of hormones.

2. About twenty minutes before the hot flash, your body's core temperature begins to rise.

3. Your heart starts pumping faster to rush blood to the surface of your skin. As your blood pressure increases, you may feel dizzy, anxious, weak, or nauseated.

Help for Hot Flashes

Try these six strategies if you find yourself getting flashed:

Identify your hot spots. Keep a record of when and where your hot flashes occur. Look for patterns, then try to avoid potential triggers. Likely culprits are stress, spicy foods, hot drinks, caffeine, alcoholic beverages, and cigarette smoking.

Get moving. Studies have shown that regular physical activity can help stop hot flashes cold. In one study of more than 1,600 women from the University of Newcastle in Callaghan, Australia, sedentary women were twice as likely to have hot flashes as their more physically active counterparts. The Fit and Sexy program gets you up and moving to ensure that you have as few flashes as possible!

Drink up. The moment you feel a hot flash coming on, try downing eight ounces of cold water to lower your body temperature.

Dress in layers. If you dress in layers, you can easily remove pieces of clothing when you feel a flash coming on.

Get to the point. Research suggests that acupuncture can help minimize hot flashes, as well as provide relief for other menopausal symptoms.

Turn down the heat. To combat night sweats, lower your thermostat to 64°F or less, put a fan near your bed, sleep on a towel, and keep a bottle of cold water on your nightstand.

4. Your skin temperature increases between one and seven degrees Fahrenheit.

5. You feel hot, hot, hot, mostly in your head, face, neck, and upper body.

6. Your blood vessels expand and warm blood rushes to the surface of your skin. This could result in a flushed look.

7. Your sweat glands start pumping to cool off your body.

8. The sweat evaporates, causing you to lose some of your body heat. You may experience a chill.

9. Your body temperature gradually returns to normal.

10. Average time of this event: 3.5 minutes, but it can last anywhere from thirty seconds to one hour.

11. Average number of flashes per day: three to four.

12. Most common times to experience hot flashes: between 6:00 and 8:00 a.m. and between 6:00 and 10:00 p.m.

Be Still My Beating Heart

Remember back in high school, when your heart would start pounding whenever you laid eyes on your secret crush? Unfortunately, the heart palpitations that can accompany perimenopause—and often occur in conjunction with hot flashes—are the result of hormonal fluctuations, not love.

No doubt, it can be disconcerting to feel your heart suddenly go into overdrive or skip a beat. But in all likelihood, there's no reason to worry. Heart palpitations can be a normal occurrence during menopause, when your hormones are going haywire. However, if they persist, you should consult your doctor, as they could signal a health problem such as thyroid disease, anemia, or hypoglycemia.

If the palpitations come with dizziness, fainting, shortness of breath, or tightness in the chest, you should get a cardiac evaluation as soon as possible. If you're postmenopausal, you're at higher risk of heart disease, so you should seek immediate medical attention for any heart irregularities.

If and when a heart palpitation does strike, be sure to sit down and breathe deeply until your pulse returns to normal. It's also smart to avoid stimulants such as alcholic beverages, nicotine, caffeine, and decongestants, which can exacerbate your symptoms.

The Moody Blues

If the other side effects of menopause don't rock your world, the crazy mood swings certainly might. That's what happened to my friend Kelly, a forty-eight-year-old nurse practitioner who lives in my neighborhood. Her temperament has always been very even keeled. But then perimenopause hit her like a Category Five hurricane.

At first, when she started feeling edgy, she thought it might be a bad case of PMS. But then she didn't get her period, and the irritability continued for months and months. She now describes it as an emotional firestorm. She lost all of her patience with her husband and kids, and would fly off the handle at the slightest provocation. At other times, she would just cry and cry. One night, she remembers sobbing while watching a heart-wrenching segment of the nightly news, then getting so riled up about another news item that she felt like throwing something. She thought she was losing it.

Experts aren't exactly certain what causes the emotional volatility that affects at least 15 percent of perimenopausal women. Some believe that decreasing levels of estrogen and other hormones prompt the brain to produce less serotonin, which regulates mood. Others feel that the

Thyroid 411

You hear about it all the time, but what exactly is your thyroid? It's a gland located at the base of your neck that regulates cell metabolism, or the rate at which cells grow and die. As part of this process, your thyroid helps determine how fast your body expends energy in the form of calories. In that respect, it can have a big impact on your waistline.

Occasionally, though, your thyroid can malfunction, causing your metabolism to get out of whack. With hyperthyroidism, the thyroid produces excess amounts of hormones that speed up many of the body's functions. Unintended weight loss often accompanies an overactive thyroid. It can also cause heart palpitations, brittle hair, insomnia, and irritability. On the flip side, hypothyroidism occurs when you're not producing enough of these thyroid hormones, which can result in symptoms such as weight gain, dry skin, depression, fatigue, foggy thinking, joint pain, and muscle aches.

Thyroid disorders—especially hypothyroidism—are more common during and after menopause. An estimated 20 percent of menopausal women in the United States are diagnosed with underactive or overactive thyroids. So if you're gaining weight, your heart frequently beats rapidly, or you're always hot even when people around you are cold, don't assume that menopause is to blame.

So what do you do? Talk to your doctor. A simple blood test called a TSH (thyroid-stimulating hormone) test can diagnose high or low levels of thyroid hormone. After age fifty, this screening test is recommended every five years. Depending on your test results, your physician may prescribe medication or another form of treatment.

side effects associated with menopause, including sleep disturbances, weight gain, and fatigue, are to blame. Still others point the finger at all the pressures facing women in their forties and fifties—trying to balance our careers, marriages, children, and other responsibilities, such as the care of aging parents. Or it could be a combination of all of these.

. . . .

"I started perimenopause early, at age thirty-eight—the year that I got married. It was supposed to be the happiest time of my life. But I was crying all the time. I would just start bawling my eyes out, for no reason. I'd be skiing with my husband, and tears would be streaming out from under my goggles. I'd get so angry at myself. I felt like I was flipping out. Fortunately, my husband's a saint. It was hard on him because he didn't know what to do. But he was a rock. He really helped me get through it."

—Amy, age forty-nine

. . . .

Regardless of the reason, the impact of menopausal moodiness can be severe. It can definitely put a strain on your personal life. Research also shows that chronic stress and negativity can compromise your immune system. Studies show that a feeling of hopelessness raises your risk of developing breast cancer and lowers survival rates from it. Likewise, negative emotions appear to increase your heart attack risk. And if that isn't bad enough, stress can cause your body to release certain hormones that make you more likely to store fat.

So what's the best way to cope with the emotional roller coaster? First, remember that *this too shall pass*. There's a reason for your moodiness, and it's called hormones. And once those hormones start to stabilize, the mood swings should ease up. (Unfortunately, that could take years, so read on for some specific suggestions on how to tame your inner bitch.) Next, talk to your family, friends, and co-workers. It may help them to have some sort of explanation for your emotional state, and if they understand what you're going through, they may be more likely to give you some space, lend a helping hand, or be patient.

When it comes to your frame of mind, physical activity can be extremely beneficial. Researchers suspect that exercise increases the production of hormones known as endorphins, which helps elevate your mood and boost your energy. It may also help boost the activity of brain neurotransmitters, which are thought to help regulate emotions. Even a five-minute walk can help when you're feeling tired or irritable. It definitely works for me.

Eating small meals and snacks throughout the day can also help you control your moods. When you go without food for a long period, your serotonin levels can plummet, causing irritability. In Chapter 5, I offer other survival tips, which include opening up about your feelings. Whenever I'm going through an emotionally trying time, I like spending time with my female friends. Nothing cheers me up faster than going for a long "walk and talk" with a girlfriend—especially one who is experiencing similar difficulties and can relate.

Keep in mind: If your sadness or irritability lasts more than a few weeks or makes you feel like you can't function or get out of bed, you should consult your doctor. There's a chance that you may be experiencing clinical depression, which is best treated with a combination of medication and psychotherapy. You'll also want to rule out a thyroid condition (see page 21 for details), which also can make you feel moody and depressed.

A Senior Moment? Already?!?

If you've been having trouble remembering things lately, welcome to the club. Many women experience minor memory and concentration problems at this time of life. Most experts attribute it to normal aging, which can cause changes in our brains that make it harder to recall stored information. And then there's the sleep deprivation, fatigue, hot flashes, and other side effects that can affect our ability to think clearly.

Declining estrogen levels may be a factor as well. Estrogen receptors are present in several regions of the brain, including those involved in memory. When activated by estrogen, these receptors stimulate processes that are beneficial to the brain. They also activate levels of certain other brain chemicals implicated in memory. When estrogen levels wane, fuzzy thinking, trouble finding words, and difficulty remembering simple tasks can result.

Understandably, some women worry that these memory lapses are an early sign of Alzheimer's disease. This unspoken fear often makes them reluctant to speak up about it. However, forgetfulness is usually *not* the beginning of Alzheimer's, so try not to worry.

The good news is that the Fit and Sexy program can also help on this front, as regular exercise is one of the best ways to keep your mind sharp. When you exercise, you increase the flow of blood, oxygen, and nutrients to your brain. Exercise also helps reduce the emotional stress that can cloud your head. I know that I have my best and clearest thoughts when I'm power walking.

A wholesome diet filled with nutrients is also crucial for clear thinking and a healthy brain. Certain foods, such as blueberries and the omega-3 fatty acids found in fish, have been shown to have a positive effect on memory. More on that in Chapter 4.

Taking a Bite out of Menopause

The hormonal fluctuations associated with menopause also can affect your mouth. During perimenopause, you're more likely to experience dry mouth, bad breath, and painful, swollen, or bleeding gums. According to a study published in the *Journal of Periodontology*, at least 23 percent of women ages thirty to fifty-four end up developing an advanced state of periodontal disease, in which gum infection spreads to the ligaments and bones that support the teeth. The result is a higher risk of tooth loss and a subsequent need for dentures.

Luckily, there are some simple ways to safeguard your smile. For starters, be sure to brush and floss every day. In addition, plan to see your dentist twice a year for an exam and thorough cleaning. If you notice problems such as red, swollen, or bleeding gums, persistent bad breath, or any other unusual changes, you should check with your dentist.

Consuming enough calcium and vitamin D may help keep your jawbone strong, protecting you from tooth loss. As your dentist has undoubtedly told you, sugar erodes the surface of your teeth, increasing your risk of cavities. It also fuels the growth of plaque, which causes periodontal disease.

Et Tu, Eyesight?

During menopause, up to 50 percent of women experience *dry eyes,* which happens when your eyes don't produce enough oils and mucus to stay well lubricated. The result can be an uncomfortable scratchy feeling and teary eyes. Over-the-counter moisturizing eyedrops can help remedy the problem. You also may want to try using a cool-mist humidifier to keep more moisture in the air.

Floaters are more likely to appear during and after the menopausal years. They're essentially tiny particles that float around within the vitreous—a gelatin-like substance that fills the inside of your eye. This creates small specks in your field of vision, which you're most likely to notice when looking at a solid background, such as a blank wall or the sky. Although they are annoying, floaters are harmless and tend to go away over time.

Cataracts are also a growing threat as you age. They can develop when clumps of protein accumulate in the lens of your eye, reducing the amount of light that reaches your retina. Another type of cataract occurs when the lens of your eye slowly becomes a yellowish-brownish color. As the cataracts gradually grow in size, your vision can become cloudy or blurred, or it may acquire a brownish tint. Ultimately, cataracts can interfere with your daily activities, such as reading and driving. Fortunately, simple surgery can be done to remove them and restore your vision.

An even more serious concern after menopause is *age-related macular degeneration*—a condition that causes mild to severe vision loss in millions of Americans each year. It occurs when tissue in the macula, the part of your retina that's responsible for central vision, deteriorates, causing blurred vision or a blind spot in the center of your visual field. While it doesn't affect your peripheral vision, it can lead to severe vision loss in one or both eyes. Unlike with cataracts, vision damaged by macular degeneration can't be restored with surgery, but early detection can help minimize the damage.

Glaucoma is another thief that can steal your vision as you get older. It happens when there's too much fluid pressure in your eye, which damages your optic nerve. While there's no cure for glaucoma, medication or laser surgery can slow or even stop the progression of the disease. Without treatment, however, glaucoma can cause total and irreversible blindness.

To protect your peepers, be sure to follow these simple steps:

See an eye doctor. Routine eye exams can help catch problems such as macular degeneration and glaucoma early—the best way to prevent vision loss. Be sure to consult an ophthalmologist if you experience unusual symptoms such as blurred vision, light flashes, or eye pain. This is especially important if you're a smoker, or if you have a family history of glaucoma, diabetes, or hypertension.

Wear shades. Sunglasses can help protect you from the ultraviolet light that can harm your eyes. Look for a pair that provides at least 98 percent protection from both UVA and UVB rays.

Kick the habit. Studies show that smoking increases your chances of getting macular degeneration. Even secondary smoke may be a hazard to your eyes.

Eat your greens. Preliminary research suggests that lutein and zeaxanthin—two antioxidants found in dark green leafy vegetables, such as spinach, kale, and collard greens, as well as egg yolks and avocados—can help keep your eyes healthy.

Skin Savvy

During perimenopause, many women notice changes in their skin, including dullness, dryness, wrinkles, and uneven pigmentation. These changes are mainly the result of damage caused by sun exposure, smoking, and air pollution. But evidence also shows that declining levels of estrogen may be a factor.

Estrogen is believed to influence the production of collagen, the connective tissue that keeps your skin looking plump, firm, and smooth. According to some estimates, skin loses up to 30 percent of its collagen in the first five years after menopause. In addition, oil glands tend to decrease their secretions, resulting in dryness, and cell renewal slows down, causing our complexions to lose their luster. Skin spots, lesions, and skin cancers also increase with age.

Fortunately, we can do a great deal to preserve the health of our skin and possibly even reverse some of the damage that has already been done. The first line of defense is reducing your exposure to the sun. I'll confess: I was guilty of sunbathing in my teens and twenties. But these days, I rarely leave home without wearing sunblock with an SPF of 30 or higher, especially on my face and neck. When I first moved to Los Angeles and started working with famous actresses and models such as Penelope Ann Miller, Julianne Phillips, and Claudia Schiffer, I couldn't help but notice that they had very smooth, porcelain complexions. I also noticed that whenever they went outside, they would slather on sunblock and wear big hats. It made me realize that you must take precautions if you want skin that looks as young and beautiful as theirs.

Exercise can also help restore your youthful glow by boosting your blood circulation and helping you sleep better. Again, this is another benefit of the Fit and Sexy program. To keep your skin hydrated, so it doesn't look dry and flaky, you'll also want to drink plenty of water. If you're like me, you may get bored drinking plain water. In Chapter 4, I'll share my favorite ways for sneaking in eight or more glasses a day, including fun, colorful ice cubes.

. . . .

"Perimenopause wasn't fun. Instead of my periods getting lighter, I had heavy bleeding and really bad cramps, which lasted for about four or five years. So it was a relief when I finally stopped menstruating. There was a freedom involved, and I didn't have to worry about carrying tampons or sanitary napkins anymore. I was happy to be done with it."

—Marsha, age sixty-two

. . . .

As you may know, a number of new skin treatments can help reduce the visible signs of aging. To combat wrinkles, skin care specialist Nerida Joy, who has worked with Courteney Cox and Jennifer Garner and has been my personal skin guru for fifteen years, recommends the regular use of topical creams designed to work on the dermis—the layer of skin beneath the epidermis that contains sebaceous glands, blood vessels, and collagen. These include products containing ingredients such as peptides, alpha lipoic acid, DMAE, alpha hydroxy acids, and hyaluronic acid. To minimize brown spots and soften wrinkles, you could try small amounts of Retin-A, a vitamin A derivative, or alpha arbutin, which is considered safer than hydroquinone-based skin lighteners, Joy explains. In addition, laser treatments can help even up your skin tone, but you shouldn't do more than two or three consecutive sessions, Joy says. Talk to your dermatologist to find out which products and procedures may work best for you.

When it comes to your skin, hormone therapy may offer some advantages as well. In one small study conducted at Yale University, combined HT (a mix of estrogen and progestin) was associated with fewer wrinkles and better skin elasticity. In the study, researchers compared nine post-menopausal women undergoing long-term hormone therapy with eleven postmenopausal women who weren't taking hormones. Their conclusion: Although HT can't reverse skin damage, it may stop some new wrinkles from developing.

Headache SOS

Some research shows that perimenopausal hormonal changes may play a role in headaches. While some women report fewer headaches and migraines, others find that their symptoms increase in frequency or severity. Migraines have been shown to be a side effect of hormone therapy. Sleep deprivation and stress, which are common among perimenopausal women, may also increase your risk.

You can do a number of things if headaches or migraines are interfering with your day-to-day functioning. Start by trying to pinpoint possible triggers. In a notebook, write down the time and date of each headache or migraine, along with details about your food intake, exercise, sleep habits, and stress levels for that day. Note what the headache felt like. Where was it located? How long did it last? How severe was it? After a few weeks, review the log and look for patterns.

In addition, you may want to avoid certain foods and drinks that can cause headaches and migraines, including cured meats such as ham and bologna, aged cheeses, monosodium glutamate (MSG), and alcohol (especially red wine).

Stress has been shown to bring on headaches. If you ask me, nothing's more effective than exercise for reducing tension. When I'm feeling stressed, I especially love going for a walk outdoors or taking a soothing yoga class. In Chapter 5, I'll discuss some of my other ideas for keeping stress at a minimum.

Some women manage their headache and migraine pain with over-the-counter medicines such as ibuprofen (Advil or Motrin) or acetaminophen (Tylenol)—but be sure to limit your intake if you regularly consume three or more alcoholic beverages a day. If not, some prescription medications, including oral triptans (Zomig, Maxalt, Imitrex) and combination migraine drugs, may do the trick.

If your headaches or migraines are very frequent or severe, or if they strike on a regular basis, be sure to see your doctor or a neurologist. In all likelihood, nothing is seriously wrong. But it's always better to be safe than sorry.

Let's Talk about Sex

When I started writing this book, I asked some of my close friends about how perimenopause had affected their sex life. The general response was, "What sex life?!?" There are definitely times that I can relate. After all, between our careers and families and all our other responsibilities, who has the time and energy for a roll in the hay?

But for some women, the time crunch isn't the only issue. During menopause, hormonal changes can cause the vulva and vagina walls to become thin, dry, and less elastic, making intercourse uncomfortable or even painful. Factor in other side effects such as weight gain, hot flashes, fatigue, and lack of sleep, and it's no great shock that between 20 and 45 percent of menopausal women experience a loss of libido.

If you find yourself experiencing vaginal dryness, you can try some simple—and discreet—solutions. For example, taking a warm bath before intercourse may make sex more comfortable and enjoyable. Over-the-counter water-based lubricants, such as K-Y Jelly's new Warming Liquid Personal Lubricant, can provide temporary relief. Or try a vaginal moisturizer, such as Replens Long-Lasting Vaginal Moisturizer, which has been shown to be as effective as estrogen creams in restoring moisture to the vagina.

Some scientific evidence shows that hormone therapy (either combined HT or estrogen only) can be effective in treating moderate to severe vaginal dryness. But first you may want to ask your ob-gyn about prescription vaginal estrogen creams, the vaginal estrogen ring, and low doses of estrogen in the form of pills or patches, which can help enhance vaginal lubrication. Because the estrogen dose is small, they're considered less risky than taking hormones.

An Urgent Matter

Of all the uncomfortable problems that can accompany menopause, *urinary incontinence*—involuntary leakage of urine—may be the most dreaded. It can happen for a number of reasons. To begin with, decreased estrogen can cause your bladder to weaken and the lining of your urethra (the passageway through which urine exits your bladder) to thin. Other factors, including childbirth (especially vaginal deliveries), gynecologic surgery, and being overweight, can also increase your risk.

There are two main types of incontinence. With *stress incontinence*, small amounts of urine may leak out when you cough, laugh, sneeze, or do activities (such as jogging or weight lifting) that put pressure on your bladder. With *urge incontinence*, also known as *overactive bladder*, you can lose larger amounts of urine at any time, for no identifiable reason.

Incontinence can be an embarrassing problem that affects your way of life—whether it requires staying close to a bathroom, wearing special panty liners, or avoiding activities that you enjoy. But it isn't something that you just have to live with. Simple exercises—known as Kegels—can help fight both kinds of incontinence by strengthening your pelvic floor muscles. If you have stress incontinence, you can also try losing weight, quitting smoking, and avoiding caffeinated beverages.

If lifestyle changes don't work, ask your physician about other treatments, including bladder training, electrical stimulation, and biofeedback. Surgery can be very successful in alleviating stress incontinence as well. Or, if you have urge incontinence, there are medications that may help.

Oh, My Achy Joints!

If you don't already feel over the hill, the joint pain and stiffness that's common during and after menopause is bound to make you feel your age. The clinical name for it is *osteoarthritis,* and it's a by-product of wear and tear, but the condition can be exacerbated by a lack of estrogen in the body.

Osteoarthritis occurs when the cartilage that covers the ends of your bones breaks down. As a result, your bones rub together, causing pain, swelling, and loss of mobility. With osteoarthritis, the pain is usually focused in weight-bearing joints, such as your hips, knees, and lower back, or your fingers and toes. You're most likely to feel it when you get up in the morning or after using a particular joint for a long period of time.

Low-impact aerobic exercise, such as walking, cycling, and swimming, is one of the best ways to combat osteoarthritis. It can help alleviate the pain and stiffness that can get worse with inactivity. Likewise, strength training can help by developing the muscles that protect and support your joints.

Excess body weight can place stress on your joints, causing them to wear out faster—another reason to shed any extra pounds that you're carrying. My Fit and Sexy formula of regular cardio and resistance exercise, combined with healthy eating, is a proven recipe for permanent weight loss.

An Affair of the Heart

Your heart is your life source. This powerful muscle acts as a pump, sending oxygen-rich blood to nourish other parts of your body. When you're young, your female hormones, including estrogen, serve as your heart protector. These hormones control the amount of fat, also called *lipids,* in your body, arming you against heart attacks and strokes. Lipids make up the cholesterol in your bloodstream.

During and after menopause, when our estrogen levels drop, our ability to regulate our lipid levels decreases. The result? A thickening of the arteries with fatty deposits that inhibit blood from pumping easily through our blood vessels to our hearts. According to the American Heart Association (AHA), more than half of all women over age fifty die from heart disease (that's more than men)—nearly twice as many as succumb to all the different forms of cancer combined.

What can you do? Be proactive. Starting at age forty-five, get your cholesterol and triglyceride levels checked—otherwise known as a lipid profile—every five years. A total cholesterol level of less than 200 is considered desirable. Optimally, your LDL or "bad" cholesterol should be 130 or less, and your HDL or "good" cholesterol should be 50 or higher. Your triglycerides should be 150 or lower, or preferably around 75. If your numbers don't measure up, your doctor may prescribe a cholesterol-lowering medication along with exercise and dietary modifications.

It's also important to keep tabs on your blood pressure. It's been estimated that 20 percent or more of North American women ages forty-five to sixty-four have mild to severe high blood pressure—a major risk factor for heart attacks and strokes. Ideally, according to the AHA, your blood pressure should be less than 120/80. If you fall in the normal

Six Tips to Take to Heart

Be a loser. Excess body fat, especially in the abdominal region, is associated with a higher risk of heart attack and stroke. To minimize your risk, you should have a body mass index (BMI) of less than 25, and a waist circumference of less than 35 inches. To calculate your BMI, multiply your weight in pounds by 703, divide by your height in inches, then divide again by your height in inches. To determine your waist circumference, put a tape measure around the largest part of your waist.

Curb your cocktails. Light to moderate alcohol intake (about 5 fluid ounces of wine, a 12-ounce beer, or 1.5 ounces of 80-proof liquor a day) has been shown to increase HDL levels and lower blood pressure. But tipping the bottle any more ups your risk for cardiovascular disease.

Stop puffing. Smoking raises blood pressure and narrows arteries, which increases the likelihood of suffering a heart attack or stroke—not to mention lung cancer, osteoporosis, emphysema, and periodontal disease.

Shake the salt habit. To prevent high blood pressure, experts advise middle-aged women to limit sodium intake to 1,500 milligrams a day—just a little more than a half teaspoon of table salt.

Control your blood sugar. Diabetes—a condition in which your body can't regulate the amount of glucose (sugar) in your blood—significantly increases your risk for heart disease to three to seven times the rate for those without diabetes. Why? Diabetes prevents the growth of new blood vessels in the heart and damages already existing blood vessels. If you have diabetes, you already know how to control your blood sugar, and hopefully you're doing so. For many, their diabetes goes undiagnosed. If you've reached age forty-five, talk to your doctor about taking a fasting blood glucose test to look for elevated blood sugar levels. This test should be done every three years. We all need to watch our sugar intake. Be aware of how much you're consuming and try to cut back on sugary foods.

range, the AHA recommends getting tested every three years. For mild hypertension, your physician may propose lifestyle modifications, such as losing weight, exercising, and cutting back on salt. For severe high blood pressure, a hypertension medication may be recommended.

Experts have long known that physical activity is good for your heart. And you don't need to run marathons to get the benefits. In fact, a recent study indicates that smaller amounts of moderate-intensity exercise—such as going for a brisk, three-mile walk about four times a week—can significantly reduce your risk of cardiovascular disease. While the researchers emphasize that more exercise is better, I think it's great to know that even a quick power walk can help protect your ticker.

While hormone therapy (both combined HT and estrogen only) was once thought to protect against heart attack and stroke, the latest research shows that it may actually increase your risk slightly. So if you have risk factors for heart disease, you may be better off staying off hormones.

While the statistics are alarming, you have the power to keep yourself from becoming one of the numbers. Watch your diet. Exercise. Get regular medical checkups. And follow the other guidelines listed on page 34.

Boning Up on Osteoporosis

The decline in estrogen production associated with menopause can pack a one-two punch on our bones. In the years immediately following menopause, many women experience rapid bone loss, which then slows but can continue through the postmenopausal years. This loss of bone can lead to osteoporosis. According to the American College of Obstetricians and Gynecologists (ACOG), about 13 to 18 percent of American women age fifty or older have osteoporosis, and an additional 37 to 50 percent have *osteopenia*—mild bone loss that is often the precursor to osteoporosis.

Often called the bone thief, osteoporosis is like a burglar that sneaks into your home while you're out. You don't see or hear it, but the results can be devastating. If left untreated, the disease can progress silently until bones become fragile and break. At greatest risk are bones in your hips, spine, and wrists. Spinal fractures can cause severe back pain, loss of height, and a curved spine, while a hip fracture can impair your ability to walk unassisted and often requires major surgery.

Calcium is an indispensable nutrient for bone health. For that reason, experts from the National Institutes of Health recommend consuming at least 1,000 milligrams of calcium a day if you're under age fifty. If you're over age fifty, aim for at least 1,000 milligrams daily if you're taking hormones, and 1,500 milligrams if you're not. In Chapter 4, you'll find a list of the best food sources, along with tips such as the optimum time of day to pop a supplement. You should also be sure to get enough vitamin D, because it helps your body absorb calcium. Recommended daily intakes are 200 IU for women under age fifty, and 400 IU for women over age fifty. While your body can obtain vitamin D from food, an even better source is sunlight, as your skin produces it when exposed to ultraviolet light. On page 161, I'll explain how long to stay in the sun without sunscreen to get a sufficient dose.

Just as a muscle gets stronger the more you use it, a bone becomes stronger and denser when you place demands on it. A lack of exercise, particularly as you get older, may contribute to lower bone mass or density. However, two types of exercise can help you maintain or even increase bone health: weight-bearing and resistance exercise. Weight-bearing activities require your muscles to work against gravity; they include walking, jogging, stair climbing, and jumping rope. Also effective are resistance exercises designed to build strength and muscle mass, such as using free weights and weight machines found at gyms and health clubs. My Fit and Sexy program involves a combination of both types.

One known risk factor for osteoporosis is smoking. I know that you've been told this a million times, but if you're still lighting up, it's

Should You Get Tested for Osteoporosis?

The American College of Obstetricians and Gynecologists (ACOG) recommends that all postmenopausal women age sixty-five or older be routinely screened for osteoporosis. ACOG advises that bone mineral density (BMD) testing is also appropriate for the following groups:

- Individuals exposed to certain drugs and substances (such as cigarette tobacco, lithium, and heparin) associated with an increased risk of osteoporosis.

- Pre- and postmenopausal women with certain diseases or medical conditions associated with an increased risk of osteoporosis, including endometriosis, hemophilia, lymphoma, leukemia, eating and nutritional disorders, rheumatoid arthritis, and multiple sclerosis.

- Postmenopausal women who have one or more risk factors, including a family history of osteoporosis, being of Caucasian race, low weight and body mass index, poor nutrition, an inactive lifestyle, low lifetime calcium intake, cigarette smoking, alcoholism, early menopause, and estrogen deficiency.

- All postmenopausal women who have sustained a fracture as an adult.

If you fall into any of these categories, talk to your doctor about getting a baseline screening for osteoporosis. Unless you develop more risk factors, such as a bone fracture, you can limit follow-up tests to every two years.

---

time to quit. And while light to moderate drinking (about 5 fluid ounces of wine, 12 ounces of beer, or 1.5 ounces of 80-proof liquor a day) may benefit your heart, it isn't good for your bones. In fact, consuming more than 7 ounces of alcohol a week has been shown to lower bone density and increase your risk of fractures.

All postmenopausal women over age sixty-five, and those with at least one risk factor for osteoporosis, should have their bone mineral density tested on a routine basis. (See "Should You Get Tested for Osteoporosis?" on page 37.) The standard screening test involves a form of X-ray technology called dual-energy X-ray absorptiometry (DEXA), a quick, painless procedure that usually takes between ten and thirty minutes. Because low-dose X-rays are used, the exposure to radiation is limited.

Hormone therapy (either combination HT or estrogen only) has been shown to have a positive effect on bone density—though the protection only lasts as long as you're taking it. But before going on hormones, you should investigate other treatment options for osteoporosis, including drugs called bisphosphates (such as Fosamax and Actonel) and selective estrogen receptor modulators (SERMs), some of which may protect against breast cancer. These medications don't have the same health risks as HT; however, they can come with unpleasant side effects, such as heartburn and constipation.

Staying Abreast of Breast Cancer

Unfortunately, as for heart disease, the risk of getting breast cancer goes up as we get older, with most cases of breast cancer occurring in women over age sixty. Although we all know women who've been diagnosed under age forty, breast cancer is uncommon before menopause. Generally, breast cancer rates begin to increase after age forty and peak in women age seventy and older.

Why the change? According to some experts, it's back to the hormones. High levels of estrogen after menopause may cause cells in the breast to become cancerous. In fact, women who go through menopause at a later age than usual have a higher risk of breast cancer. Why? It's simple math. The later your menopause, the longer you've had estrogen circulating in your body.

It's scary, I know, but you can protect yourself. First and foremost, get your mammograms. The American Cancer Society recommends that you get a mammography screening every year beginning at age forty. For those of you who haven't had one, the procedure—which takes only about thirty minutes—uses low-dose radiation to examine breast tissue for tumors and other irregularities. According to a recent study in the *New England Journal of Medicine,* from 1990 to 2000 the death rate from breast cancer dropped by about 24 percent for women ages thirty to seventy-nine. Researchers attribute nearly half the drop to mammogram screenings, and the other half to better treatments.

An estimated 15 percent of tumors aren't caught by mammography, but can be felt. That's why many health organizations continue to encourage annual breast exams from a qualified health professional. Most gynecologists perform one at your yearly checkup. Your doctor will look for lumps and changes in size and shape, not just in your breasts but over the entire chest area and from your armpit to your collarbone. Tell your doctor about any concerns you may have if you've noticed differences.

For years, monthly breast self-exams were considered a "must" in the fight against breast cancer. But recently, the American Cancer Society and other organizations have backed off from that advice. That's because of new research showing that self-exams aren't so effective in catching early cancers. However, self-exams still may offer a benefit—namely, by making you more familiar with your breasts, so you'll notice any changes, if they develop.

While some of the risk factors for breast cancer—such as a family history of the disease, being of Caucasian race, and being over age sixty—are beyond your control, others *can* be managed. For example, you're more likely to develop breast cancer if you're overweight or obese. Experts aren't entirely sure why, but one theory is that excess body fat boosts estrogen levels and other hormones that speed the growth of tumors. The good news is, by losing just five or ten pounds, you can reduce your risk.

Physical inactivity is another risk factor for breast cancer. In one recent study published in the *Journal of the American Medical Association*, women who walked just three hours a week at an average pace of 2 to 2.9 miles per hour cut their risk of dying from breast cancer in half.

. . . .

"Perimenopause was a real emotional roller coaster for me. I felt totally out of balance. For the first couple years, I used exercise to manage my moods. But after a while, it wasn't enough. So I talked to my gynecologist, and she made me realize that I needed more help. She recommended psychotherapy and got me started on low-dose estrogen therapy. There's breast cancer in my family. But she told me there's no conclusive evidence that estrogen therapy feeds breast tumors. Ultimately, I decided that the benefits outweighed the risks. It's really important for me to keep myself mentally healthy through this period. The estrogen therapy, along with the exercise and psychotherapy, has really helped me keep my life on an even keel."

—Nathalie, age fifty-two

. . . .

Those nightly cocktails, while they can be relaxing, may also be bad for your breasts. According to the ongoing Nurses' Health Study at Harvard University, women who have one drink or more per day have a 60 percent higher risk of developing breast cancer than women who don't drink. Exactly why this occurs isn't known, but it may be because alcohol raises the level of estrogen in your body.

And if you're considering hormones, take note: According to the latest research, combined hormone therapy raises your risk for breast cancer slightly, and the risk increases the longer you stay on it. (Estrogen-only therapy, on the other hand, appears to be safe.) So if you're at high risk for breast cancer, or have a personal or family history of the disease, you'll want to think twice about combination HT.

The Skinny on Hormone Therapy

If you're confused about whether to take hormones, it's no wonder. For more than sixty years, doctors have been prescribing them in different forms to manage menopausal symptoms, including hot flashes and vaginal dryness. In the mid-1980s, after researchers found that estrogen could help slow bone loss, the Food and Drug Administration (FDA) approved it to treat osteoporosis. For a time, experts suspected that hormone therapy (HT) could protect women from heart disease, too. But in recent years, two large-scale studies have questioned its safety, leaving many of us—including me—wondering what to do.

The first concerns about hormone replacement were raised back in the 1970s. That's when researchers discovered that estrogen stimulated the lining of the uterus, putting women at high risk of uterine cancer. To counter these effects, doctors started adding another hormone, progesterone, to the mix. This estrogen-progestin combination soon became standard fare for women who still had a uterus. Estrogen alone continued to be used for those who had undergone a hysterectomy.

Then, in 2002 and 2004, came a bombshell: the findings from the Women's Health Initiative (WHI), a major, fifteen-year research program sponsored by the National Institutes of Health (NIH). The study, which involved more than 161,000 postmenopausal women between ages fifty and seventy-nine, was designed to determine to what extent hormone therapy (both combined estrogen-progestin and estrogen only) protected women against heart disease. It also examined how HT increased or decreased the risk of other serious health problems, including breast cancer, bone fractures, colon cancer, and dementia.

One part of the study, which included sixteen thousand women taking standard-dose combination HT, was supposed to last eight years. Investigators hoped it would yield definitive answers on the benefits of HT. It didn't work out that way. After a little more than five years, researchers halted the study after finding that women taking combined estrogen-progestin were more likely to experience heart attacks, strokes, breast cancer, and blood clots compared with those on a placebo. On the positive side, they had fewer spine and hip fractures and were less likely to develop colon cancer. But as far as the WHI researchers were concerned, the downsides outweighed the benefits.

Two years later, in 2004, a second arm of the WHI study, which followed almost eleven thousand postmenopausal women without a uterus taking estrogen only, was also halted early. Like the estrogen-progestin combo, estrogen-only therapy was found to slightly increase a woman's risk of blood clots and strokes. However, it wasn't associated with a higher risk of heart disease or breast cancer, and was shown to reduce the risk of hip fractures.

The announcement of these discoveries and the suspension of the WHI studies sent shock waves through the medical community. Doctors across the country began calling their patients and advising them to stop HT immediately. Almost overnight, the standard recommendations for HT usage changed drastically. Before, it wasn't unusual for physicians to prescribe long-term HT to prevent heart disease and bone loss as well as relieve acute symptoms, and many women had been taking hormones for decades. Now, most recommend HT only for short-term relief of severe menopausal symptoms.

Since then, two new studies have shed new light on some of the original WHI findings. The first, based on the well-established Harvard Nurses' Health Study and published in the *Journal of Women's Health*, found that women who began hormone therapy (either estrogen only or combination estrogen-progestin) at or near the onset of menopause had about a 30 percent *lower* risk for heart disease than women who didn't use HT. By comparison, older women who started HT at least ten years past menopause didn't seem to experience any heart benefits or risks.

The second study, published in the *Archives of Internal Medicine*, examined the data on women from the second arm of the WHI study, who took estrogen only. It showed that those who started estrogen therapy between ages fifty and fifty-nine had a 45 percent *lower* risk for bypass surgery and angioplasty. Those who started taking estrogen between ages sixty and sixty-nine, on the other hand, didn't experience the same protection, and women who began after age seventy had an 11 percent higher risk of heart attack.

The bottom line? When it comes to hormones, experts now believe that timing could be key. In other words, if you start HT before or soon after menopause, you're likely to face fewer risks and more benefits. However, until we know more, you aren't advised to take hormones to prevent heart disease. And while hormones may help your heart and your bones, they could put you at higher risk for blood clots and, possibly, breast cancer.

Likewise, the WHI studies looked only at specific doses of estrogen or estrogen-progestin taken orally. Some experts have speculated that women may be able to avoid many of the health risks by taking smaller doses or using other delivery methods, such as skin patches and creams. But more research is needed before we have clear answers.

Are Hormones Right for You?

Good question, and one that you must discuss with your doctor. If your symptoms are disrupting your life—and can't be managed through exercise and diet—hormone therapy may be worth considering. But before moving forward, you need to weigh the potential benefits and risks based on your personal and family health history. So talk to your physician about your symptoms, as well as your risk factors for heart disease,

Who Should Consider Hormone Therapy?

Whether to take hormones is a personal decision that you should make based on your individual health history as well as the nature and severity of your perimenopausal symptoms. So talk to your doctor about your symptoms as well as your risk factors. While it shouldn't be a substitute for your physician's advice, this chart can help you determine whether hormone therapy might be right for you.

You may be a candidate for combined hormone therapy if:

- Perimenopausal symptoms, such as hot flashes, mood swings, and vaginal dryness, are making you miserable.
- You've tried exercising and changing your diet, but nothing seems to help.
- You haven't reached menopause yet.
- You still have a uterus.
- You don't have a history of strokes, blood clots, or breast cancer.

You may be a candidate for estrogen-only therapy if:

- Perimenopausal symptoms, such as hot flashes, mood swings, and vaginal dryness, are making you miserable.
- You've tried exercising and changing your diet, but nothing seems to help.
- You haven't reached menopause yet.
- You don't have a uterus.
- You don't have a history of blood clots or strokes.

Hormone therapy (either combined or estrogen only) probably isn't for you if:

- You have hardly any perimenopausal symptoms, or your symptoms are mild.

- You're plagued by hot flashes or other side effects, but you haven't tried managing them with lifestyle changes, such as exercise or watching your diet.

- You have a personal or family history of blood clots or strokes.

- You haven't had a period in more than five to ten years.

breast cancer, osteoporosis, and other illnesses. And don't leave anything out! Your doctor needs full information to help you make the best decision.

I've been lucky so far; with the exception of some wicked mood swings, I haven't been plagued by uncomfortable perimenopausal symptoms—at least not yet. So it's hard for me to imagine taking hormones. Besides, I'm wary of putting anything into my system that might affect other bodily functions. In general, when it comes to medication, I tend to be an old-fashioned girl. From pregnancy to PMS, exercise and nutritious eating have helped me through many hormonally charged times. So for now, I plan to tackle perimenopause the all-natural way.

Natural Remedies, Herbs, and Other Holistic Helpers

When you walk into a health food store, a pharmacy, or even the supermarket, you may find yourself bombarded with supplements, herbs, and other products promising you the moon. Buyer beware, says the American College of Obstetricians and Gynecologists (ACOG). For most of these products, testing, if any, has been limited and results are often inconclusive. Also, they aren't strictly regulated by the FDA or any other government agency. So you can't be sure what you're getting when you buy them.

Consider that a review of ginseng products conducted by the American Botanical Council showed that 60 percent of the products contained little ginseng and 25 percent contained no ginseng at all. Even worse, many were heavily laden with caffeine. That's pretty scary, especially when you consider that caffeine can aggravate some of the symptoms of menopause, including anxiety, irritability, and mood swings.

With that said, many women—including friends and clients of mine—turn to botanicals for the treatment of their menopausal symptoms. Here are some of the most popular ones and what we know about them:

Soy protein and isoflavones, the two main components of soybeans, have estrogen-like properties that may help ease some menopausal symptoms, particularly hot flashes. While considered safe in moderate amounts, consumption of large quantities of soy protein or isoflavones—whether from whole foods or supplements—could be risky, especially for women with a history of breast cancer and other estrogen-dependent cancers. So enjoy soy, but don't go overboard.

Black cohosh (also known as black snakeroot, squaw root, or bugbane) comes from the root of a wildflower. It is the leading herbal remedy sold in Europe to relieve menopausal symptoms, including hot flashes, vaginal dryness, sleep disturbances, and depression. Exactly how it works in the body is unclear, but it may stimulate the ovaries to increase estrogen production. The most well-known brand is Remifemin. In one study in the March 2002 issue of the *Journal of Women's Health and Gender-Based Medicine,* most women reported a 70 percent decrease in physical and emotional symptoms, including hot flashes and irritability, when they took the standard dose of Remifemin (40 milligrams per day) for twelve weeks. According to some experts, however, it shouldn't be used for longer than six months, or along with estrogen therapy or blood pressure medications.

Dong quai (Chinese angelica, tang-kuei, dang-gui), which comes from the root of a flowering plant, has been used in China for more than 1,200 years. It is thought to help regulate menstrual periods and ease cramps and menopausal symptoms. However, in a clinical trial of seventy-one women published in the journal *Fertility and Sterility,* it was found to be no more effective than a placebo in reducing hot flashes. Critics of the study have noted that the daily dose used in the study (4.5 grams) was lower than that often used in traditional Chinese medicine. They also contend that dong quai is never used alone, as it was in this study, and that botanicals must be taken together in a balanced formula to have effects on menopausal symptoms.

Because it can trigger heavy uterine bleeding, dong quai shouldn't be used by anyone taking anticlotting drugs or by women with fibroids, hemophilia, and other blood-clotting disorders.

Evening primrose oil (also called evening star) comes from seeds rich in gamma linolenic acid (GLA). As oils, capsules, and tinctures to tea, it is thought to help relieve menopausal symptoms, including hot flashes and breast tenderness. But once again, the scientific evidence doesn't support these claims. Women with epilepsy and serious mental health disorders, as well as those taking anticlotting or antianxiety medications, shouldn't take it.

Ginseng (Panax ginseng) is commonly used in Chinese medicine to fight fatigue and boost immunity. However, no strong research supports this notion. In fact, studies have shown that ginseng doesn't relieve hot flashes. In fact, in 1999, when Ginsana, the largest manufacturer of ginseng, funded a study of 384 women to investigate the effects of ginseng in menopausal women, no differences were found between those taking ginseng and those given placebos. The women took either Ginsana, which contains 100 milligrams of the standardized ginseng extract, or an identical-looking placebo; each participant took two capsules in the morning after breakfast. Women taking the ginseng did, however, say that they were happier and that their general health was better.

Ginseng is known to have estrogen-like effects that can result in uterine bleeding. Possible side effects include high blood pressure, low blood sugar, headaches, and insomnia. Women with heart disease, diabetes, and bipolar disorder should take caution.

Wild yam, also known as Mexican yam, is an herb that contains chemicals that can be processed in a lab and changed into progesterone. Some products made with wild yam claim to have "natural progesterone" that can help relieve hot flashes and other menopausal symptoms, but no scientific evidence supports their use. In fact, some of the wild or Mexican yam creams sold at health food stores or elsewhere contain only a precursor to progesterone that is inactive when absorbed through the skin. However, certain manufacturers add synthetic progesterone to their products, which could be beneficial in terms of minimizing hot flashes—but not exactly the "natural" remedy that the package may suggest.

Chasteberry, also known as chaste tree or sage tree hemp, grows in the Mediterranean region. These reddish-brown berries look and are said to taste like peppercorns; thus, they are sometimes called monk's pepper. Some recommend it for vaginal dryness as well as for depression. Chasteberry contains hormonelike substances that produce antiandrogenic effects. In other words, it decreases levels of male hormones, and it is often recommended to reduce sex drive in males. With women, it is said to have the reverse effect on libido. Chasteberry is available in powder, tea, capsule, and liquid forms.

Natural and herbal remedies can interact with other medications, so please talk to your doctor before experimenting with any of these products. If you're already taking them, don't hide it from your physician. Full disclosure is critical to your health.

Menopause Makeover

As you can probably guess, my natural inclination and expertise favor exercise over many of the treatments mentioned here. In fact, there isn't one side effect of menopause—from mood swings to lack of energy—that exercise can't improve! In light of the mixed messages on hormone therapy, I encourage you to try my Fit and Sexy for Life program first. See how you feel. You may find that physical activity helps alleviate your hot flashes and allows you to sleep soundly through the night. My workouts and healthy eating strategies can help keep your bones strong, your cholesterol and blood pressure in check, and much, much more. Best of all, if you're smart about workouts, and build up gradually, there are no dangerous side effects! It's one of the easiest, safest, and most inexpensive ways to keep your body happy as you get older.

2

. . . .

This Is No Time
to Slow Down . . .
So Get Moving!

THOSE LOVE HANDLES, lower-body bulges, and stiff joints don't lie. Now that you're in the throes of menopause, your body is undergoing a major metamorphosis. And all of those lumps, bumps, aches, and pains are sending a clear message: It's time to get your rear in gear!

I've noticed that many women start slacking off on their workouts at this time of life—just when they need them the most. Some of them simply lose their motivation. Others think that now that they're getting older, they can start taking it easy. They feel like they don't need to push their bodies anymore. In any case, they end up doing more sitting, sitting, sitting. Over time, all that inactivity can add up to extra inches, especially around your middle.

You don't need me to explain why regular physical activity is so important. So I won't bore you by rattling on about the countless benefits. Suffice it to say that exercise is essential for a fit, firm, and healthy body. It's a proven way to protect against heart disease, cancer, osteoporosis, diabetes, and other devastating illnesses. It can help you fend off excess pounds and successfully shed the weight you may have already gained. Last but not least, it can help mitigate most menopausal symptoms, including headaches, hot flashes, irritability, and insomnia.

Even if you've been good about exercising regularly, your fitness regimen may need a tune-up. Let's be honest: what worked for you ten or twenty years ago may not be working so well now. Plus you have to take your body's current needs into account. Only doing cardio, for example, isn't going to cut it. If you're going to stay slim and healthy, you need a balanced program designed to incinerate calories and build both endurance and strength, without putting too much stress on your joints. And you should be sure to include some flexibility work, too.

. . . .

"Exercise has really helped me cope with my moods. It helps me relax and gives me an endorphin high that sticks with me through the day. It's made me stronger mentally as well as physically. When I feel strong and fit, I have more confidence and self-esteem. But mild exercise doesn't really work, at least for me. To really feel the effects, I need to break a sweat."

—Nathalie, age fifty-two

. . . .

Chances are, if you're like most women over age forty, your midsection could use some extra attention as well. To keep your waistline looking trim, you need exercises to tighten and tone your abdominal muscles.

Your core muscles are involved in almost every move that you make. By strengthening them, you can develop better balance and a more stable center of gravity. This translates to a decreased risk of injury from falling, as well as increased protection for your back.

Remember, just because you're getting older doesn't mean you have to become weak and frail. With the right fitness plan, it's possible to fight the effects of aging and gravity. You can develop strong, defined muscles. You can keep your posterior and other parts from sagging. Even better, you can build energy and stamina for your next big adventure—maybe participating in a local walk/run race, snowboarding in Aspen, or kayaking in New Zealand!

Starting today, you want to *think like an athlete*. This is what I constantly tell my forty- and fifty-something clients, and the same goes for you. What it means is treating your body with as much care as a professional athlete would. It means doing something good for it every day. It means sticking to your training program and fueling yourself with the right foods. It means acting as if it's your job. But instead of preparing for the Olympics, you're training for a long, active, and healthy life.

· ·

"To push yourself to the physical and mental limits, to ask yourself to deliver more than you think you possibly can and to come through, is the greatest high there is."

—from *A Lotus Grows in the Mud* by Goldie Hawn

· ·

Don't worry; I'm not about to tell you to spend three hours a day at the gym. In fact, as you'll discover with my Fit and Sexy plan, you can get great results in just thirty to sixty minutes a day, without ever leaving your house. But during those thirty to sixty minutes, you can't just go through the motions. If you really want to see a change in your body, you need to put as much effort as you can into your workouts. Yes, there will be some sweat involved, but believe me, it'll be worth it!

The Fit and Sexy for Life Solution

To help you stay strong, slim, and sexy through menopause and beyond, I've developed a six-day-a-week plan for blasting calories and building muscle. Here's how it works: You'll do a twenty- to thirty-minute strength routine three times a week, on Mondays, Wednesdays, and Fridays. On Tuesdays, Thursdays, and Saturdays, you'll walk and do ab exercises. At the end of each daily workout, you'll cool down with my soothing, ten-minute Stretch and Unwind routine.

I've designated Sunday as a "free" day, and I'll explain more about this on page 118. But for now, think of it as a day to do something that feels good. That could mean taking it easy or planning a fun activity with friends. It's totally up to you. If you're like me, you'll enjoy knowing that you can take a break from your workouts. It's a small "reward" that can really motivate you! Plus it can keep you from getting burned out. When Monday rolls around, you'll feel refreshed and be ready to get back to business again.

As with any fitness plan, flexibility is key to making it work. So you don't have to follow my proposed schedule to the letter. For example, you can start on a Friday instead of a Monday. You can do the cardio and/or ab work on the same day as your strength exercises. Or if you have time constraints, you can do half of your workout in the morning and half before dinner. One caveat: Don't lift weights two days in a row. That's because your muscles need a full day to recover between strength workouts.

Remember, just because you've crossed your daily workout off your list doesn't mean that you should spend the rest of the day on your butt. Every little move you make can help you boost your energy, burn more calories, and improve your health. It doesn't matter whether you're planting flowers in your garden, walking around your local mall, or vacuuming your house. So fight the urge to hit the sofa. You'll feel so much better if you keep moving. Plus research shows that even these little bits of activity can make a real difference in fending off excess pounds.

I don't want you to think of this as an exercise program. I want you to think of it as a lifestyle. In other words, these workouts shouldn't be something that you do for a few weeks or months, then stop. To get lasting benefits, you need to be consistent. Obviously, your body will reap the rewards only as long as you keep exercising. That's why I've kept it simple. To me, that's the problem with a lot of workout programs. They're so complicated or time consuming that you can't stick with them. Not so with my Fit and Sexy plan. It's so easy and straightfor-

Chaos Control

Over the years, I've observed my personal training clients closely. In the process, I've noticed that the ones who are organized are much more likely to fit exercise into their day—no matter how busy they are. As for my clients who are, shall we say, chaos queens, working out rarely happens because in their words, "there just isn't time." Nonsense. There *is* time. And there will be more time if you spend a few minutes every day getting your home, your life, and your workouts in order. Getting organized will help you feel more in control and able to tackle each day's challenges more efficiently and effectively. Here are a few tips to get you started:

Clear the clutter. Get rid of old magazines, books, clothes, appliances, and other household items that you don't use anymore. I like adhering to the one-year rule: If you haven't used it in the past year, give it away! Invest in storage containers and install shelves and hooks, so your house looks tidy and you stop wasting time digging around for things.

ward, it will become a part of your daily routine. Before you know it, you'll forget your pre–Fit and Sexy days!

Strength Train for Strong Bones and a Speedy Metabolism!

Strength training can help you achieve your best body at any time of life, but it's especially crucial now that you're getting older. As I mentioned earlier, resistance exercise is key to building strong muscles and bones, which can help stave off osteoporosis. What's more, it can help keep

Get prepared. On most mornings, I get up thirty to forty-five minutes earlier than the rest of my family to get a jump on my day. It gives me some quiet time to get organized and do some busy work, whether it's working on my newspaper column, filling out school permission slips, or paying bills. I often start by making a checklist. I write down what needs to get done, then set priorities. I decide what's most important and save my time and energy for those tasks. If you aren't a morning person, try setting aside half an hour every evening instead.

Plan your workouts. Schedule a specific time for each workout, and write it down on your calendar or plug it into your BlackBerry. Figure out what equipment you're going to need and make sure it's ready to go. For example, if your workout calls for an exercise ball and five-pound dumbbells, set them aside ahead of time. Have a CD player cued up with your favorite CDs. Or if you plan to walk on your lunch break, pack your workout clothes and sneakers into a bag, and check to make sure your iPod is charged before hitting the hay.

you free of back pain and other injuries so you stay active well into your golden years.

Strength training can also be a powerful weapon in the fight against middle-age spread. In fact, research shows that it may be just as important as cardio exercise for shedding pounds. How come? While cardio activities such as walking and jogging are great for burning calories, strength training helps you build muscle, which speeds up your metabolism—so you burn more calories all day long. According to some estimates, for every pound of muscle gained, you zap about fifty extra calories a day, which can translate to more than five pounds of body fat lost over the course of a year.

The Metabolism Connection

While your hormones may be to blame for those hot flashes and sleepless nights, another problem—a sluggish metabolism—may be causing you to pack on the pounds. That's right: in recent years, researchers have found that the weight gain that many women experience at this time of life is related to aging and inactivity, not the hormonal fluctuations that come with aging.

Our muscles are calorie-burning powerhouses. It takes more energy, in the form of calories, to sustain muscles than to sustain body fat. As we grow older and become more sedentary, we lose muscle, which causes our metabolisms to plummet. As a result, we burn fewer calories throughout the day, which, over time, can translate to extra inches.

The good news is that we can prevent and even reverse some of this muscle loss with regular exercise. While weight-bearing aerobic activities, such as walking, can help, strength training (weight lifting and other forms of exercise that involve working against resistance) is the most effective way to build muscle and keep your metabolism supercharged.

Regardless of whether you lose weight, regular strength training can help you improve your shape. Think smooth, firm, and sculpted muscles! Muscle weighs more than fat, but it takes up less space. So even if the numbers on the scale don't change, your clothes will get looser, and your body will look more firm and toned.

Strength Training 101

For maximum results—and to stay injury free—follow these simple tips.

Warm Up

Cold muscles are more susceptible to injury. So before each workout, be sure to do five minutes of light aerobic activity. You can use any piece of cardio equipment, such as a treadmill or stationary bike. Or you can go for a quick walk around the block, climb up and down stairs, or march in place.

Focus on Form

Do each exercise in a slow, controlled manner. Don't use quick, jerky movements. Make sure you can feel it in the muscles that you're trying to target.

Use Enough Resistance

To really see a change in your body, you can't just lift one-pound weights! To build muscle and boost your metabolism, you need to challenge your muscles. Be sure to get the hang of the moves—especially ones that require balance—before adding a lot of resistance. But ultimately your goal is to work your target muscles to fatigue. So if you don't feel challenged by the end of each set, you may need to switch to a heavier weight. (Recommended weight ranges are listed with each exercise.)

Listen to Your Body

If you're new to strength training or you haven't worked out in ages, be sure to take it slow and build strength gradually. Some of the moves may be difficult for you at first. But stick with it! As you get stronger and develop better balance and coordination, they *will* get easier. This program is designed to strengthen your entire body, with a special emphasis on your core and your lower body (the muscles that help support your spine and your knees). Done properly, the exercises should help prevent injuries and combat chronic knee and back pain. However, if you have an existing problem, you should consult your physician before getting started. If you experience any pain during your workout, check to make sure you're doing the exercise correctly and modify the move, if possible. If it still hurts, stop what you're doing and check with your doctor.

Walk Your Way to a Fit, Firm Body!

How do some of Hollywood's sexiest forty- and fifty-somethings, including Michelle Pfeiffer and Kim Basinger, stay in such fabulous shape? By putting one foot in front of the other. I know because I've trained many of them! While a lot of exercise fads come and go, especially in a city like Los Angeles, walking has stood the test of time, and for good reason. In addition to being a great calorie-burning workout, it can help tone and shape your muscles, strengthen your bones, and keep your heart and lungs healthy. It's also easy on your joints, and you don't need anything but a comfortable pair of shoes to do it.

Walking is one of my favorite forms of exercise. It's been a big part of my fitness regimen ever since I stopped long-distance running. About ten years ago, when I was training Meg Ryan after the birth of her son, we would run up and down the streets of Santa Monica, California. Sometimes we would go six or seven miles at a time. And it felt great! The endorphins and the feeling of sweat running down my chest gave me a natural high. These days, it's a different story. Now, thanks to sensitive joints, I can't run for miles and miles like I used to. But the good news is, I don't really need to! That's because walking can be equally effective. This may come as a surprise to many of you, but with the right walking program, you can burn just as many calories and get in great cardiovascular shape. And your joints will love you for it! Just to warn you, though: I'm not talking about some leisurely strolls in the park. I'm talking about brisk walking that really boosts your heart rate and challenges your muscles.

I love the walking program that I've put together for you. I do it now and will continue to do it for all of my days. Here's the deal: Each week, you'll do three three-mile walks. The first is a basic steady-state walk that focuses on developing speed. The second incorporates quick but intense cardio moves to really boost your heart rate. The third has some short running intervals sprinkled in to increase the intensity. Each sprint only lasts between thirty seconds and two minutes, so you won't stress your joints—and you can experience the same sense of euphoria that you get from running longer distances.

You can do all three workouts outside or inside on a treadmill. Personally, I prefer walking outdoors, where there's fresh air and changes of scenery. If you plan to do the same, you should map out a few walking routes ahead of time. Get in your car and use the odometer to clock several three-mile loops. Be sure to note where the one-mile marks are. I encourage you to vary your walking routes throughout the week. This will allow you to encounter new terrain and keep your muscles challenged. New sights and smells can also make your walks more interesting and fun.

Before you begin, be sure to invest in a good pair of walking, running, or cross-training shoes. You'll want to replace your shoes every six months or so because the treads and cushioning wear down over time. If you find a pair that you love, think about buying two of them. The shoe manufacturers change their styles so frequently that by the time you need a replacement, your favorite pair may be long gone.

Trim and Tone Your Midsection!

If you really want to know, my least favorite part of being forty-something is my poochy belly. In the past few years, every excess pound that I gain seems to go straight to my middle. Even when I'm at my ideal weight, I feel like my tummy isn't nearly as flat or toned as it was in my twenties and thirties. Oh, the joys of getting older!

But don't worry, we aren't destined to end up with menopots. With my combination of cardio exercise, strength training, and healthy eating, you can melt off the excess inches that have accumulated around your middle. In addition, to keep your midsection looking firm and slender, you'll be doing three abdominal workouts a week.

Each workout targets your four major abdominal muscles, including the rectus abdominis (the visible "six-pack" muscle), the internal and external obliques (the sides of your waist), and the transverse abdominis (the deepest abdominal muscle that helps flatten your belly). What's more, some of the moves help strengthen your erector spinae, the three pairs of muscles that run along your spine and work with your abdominal muscles to stabilize your torso and help you stand up straight.

So you really see results, I've included a variety of exercises that target your core in different ways. Believe me, these aren't your same old boring abdominal crunches. Each one has a special twist, whether it requires balance or using resistance from a weighted ball.

Many women make the mistake of not fully engaging their abs when doing core work. Therefore, they don't get the definition that they're

Working Out to *Cool Off*?

"*Exercise while I'm getting hot flashes? Not a chance!*" I can't even count how many times I have heard this from women wishing to stop their training during menopause. I understand the logic. If you are prone to sweating profusely for no reason, why would you do something that makes you sweat? But several studies have shown that hot flashes and night sweats can be eased with exercise.

In one study of 1,600 women, researchers from the University of Newcastle, Callaghan, Australia, found that sedentary women were twice as likely to report hot flashes as women who exercised. Yet another study by a team out of the University Hospital in Linkoping, Sweden, found that moderate and severe hot flashes were half as common among the physically active postmenopausal women, when compared with their more sedentary counterparts.

This may be because exercise turns off the mechanisms that elicit hot flashes. Although strenuous exercise workouts can increase body temperature, overall, active women tend to have fewer and less intense hot flashes. This may be because their bodies become more tolerant to extreme temperatures and more effective at cooling down.

---

after. Here's the trick: As you do each exercise, really focus on pulling your belly button in toward your spine, and maintain the contraction throughout the entire move. Deep breathing can help, too. Exhale on the exertion part of the exercise, and inhale as you return to the starting position.

Remember, you don't have to do hundreds of repetitions to get sexy, toned abdominals. In fact, you can get better results in fewer reps if you concentrate on keeping your core muscles engaged as you do each one. If you're doing the exercises correctly, you should be able to feel it, and you won't be able to keep going and going.

Don't Forget Your Kegels!

As we talked about earlier, a Kegel is a simple exercise designed to strengthen your pelvic floor. When done correctly and consistently, these exercises have been shown to help up to 75 percent of women overcome stress incontinence. Kegels may also enhance your sex life by increasing blood flow to your genital area and improving the muscle tone of your vagina, helping you feel more aroused and making it easier to reach orgasm.

Here's how to do them:

- Squeeze the muscles around your vaginal area as if you're trying to stop peeing midstream.

- You should feel a small lifting motion around your rectum and vagina.

- Start by holding the contraction tightly for 5 seconds, and gradually work up to 10 seconds.

- Each day, your goal should be to do 3 sets of 10 reps, allowing a 10-second rest between sets.

For best results, be sure to contract the proper muscles. Keep your abs, thighs, and buttocks relaxed; if you tighten them, you're working the wrong muscles. Some experts suggest placing a finger or two in your vagina to make sure you're squeezing in the right spot.

Kegels aren't difficult to do. The hard part, for many of us, is remembering to do them! To help remind myself, I keep a Post-it note that says "30 K's" on the dashboard of my car. Fortunately, no one else knows what it means! Alternatively, try putting a reminder on your nightstand, and do your Kegels in the morning while watching the *Today* show or before bed during a rerun of *Sex and the City*. (I'm sure Samantha would approve!)

Getting Started

OK, enough talking—it's time to start moving! If you're already active, and you don't have any injuries or major health problems, there's no reason why you can't start my Fit and Sexy program today. If you haven't exercised in the past three months, or you have high blood pressure or other serious medical conditions, talk to your doctor first.

Gear Up

To do these workouts, you'll need some basic and inexpensive tools. You can purchase most of these items at your local sporting goods store, at Target, or online at SPRI International (800-222-7774; www.spriproducts .com). Or you may be able to find secondhand equipment through the classifieds or at a garage sale right in your neighborhood.

- A medicine ball (5 pounds)

- A large exercise ball (also known as a stability ball or physioball)

- A set of dumbbells (3, 5, 8, 10, 12, and 15 pounds)

- A resistance band with handles (medium resistance)

- A weight bench or aerobics step

- A sturdy chair

- An exercise mat or towel

- A good pair of walking/running or cross-training shoes

- A stopwatch or sports watch

- A jump rope (optional)

- A pedometer (optional)

Stay Hydrated

Agua, H$_2$O, water—whatever you want to call it—just remember you need lots of it, especially when you exercise. Water helps transport oxygen to your muscles and allows you to sweat and cool off. If you aren't properly hydrated, your heart will be forced to work harder, your body is more likely to overheat, and your performance will suffer. I always keep a water bottle nearby when I'm lifting weights. When I'm out walking, I use either my CamelBak (a backpack that holds cold water and has a long straw) or a fanny pack with water bottle holders. Sipping as you go helps you maintain your hydration levels without disrupting your workout and is more effective than gulping down an entire bottle at the end. For anyone who has a hard time drinking enough plain water, I recommend trying a lightly flavored fitness water, such as Propel Fitness Water.

Pace Yourself

To get the best results, you need to put effort into your workouts and challenge your body. Your goal should be to work as hard as you comfortably can during each exercise session. But you don't want to overdo it either. If you push yourself too hard, you could end up sore or suffer an injury. So listen to your body. If you're not a regular exerciser, you may feel some discomfort, especially in the beginning. As you get in better shape, your workouts should start to feel good instead of uncomfortable. But if you experience any pain or shortness of breath, be sure to stop immediately.

Keep a Fitness Log

I've been keeping track of my workouts for longer than I can remember. In my day planner, I write down the specifics of each session—what I've done, how long I've done it, and how I felt during and afterward. Did I sweat? Was I tired or full of energy? Did it help me relax? I find it to be a great motivational tool. It creates a sense of accountability. Plus, I love looking back and seeing all I've done for my body. Similarly, it can be extremely helpful to record your daily food intake. Throughout the day, jot down what you eat, when, why, and how it made you feel. Looking back, you may see areas that need improvement, or you may realize that you're doing better than you thought. Some of my clients use their fitness logs as a way to get organized and plan their week ahead, going back each night to see if they've crossed everything off their lists. Grab your calendar or notebook and start your log tonight. I'm sure you'll find it as rewarding as I do.

Kathy's Six-Day Body Blast

Workout Schedule

Monday/Day One: Strength Workout

Tuesday/Day Two: Cardio (Core Walk) and Ab Workout

Wednesday/Day Three: Strength Workout

Thursday/Day Four: Cardio (Walk Circuit) and Ab Workout

Friday/Day Five: Strength Workout

Saturday/Day Six: Cardio (Walk/Run Intervals) and Ab Workout

Sunday/Day Seven: "Free" Day

Monday/Day One:
Strength Workout

Warm up. Start with 5 minutes of low-intensity cardio, such as walking or marching in place.

Your strength workout. Do the following exercises in the order listed. Rest 30 to 60 seconds between sets.

1. Straddle Jump Up

Stand with your feet straddling a bench. Place your hands on the bench, so you're grasping the edges of it. Keeping your hands securely on the bench, bend your knees slightly, then jump up as high as you can, landing with your feet on top of the bench. Return to the starting position. Do this for 1 minute, or as long as you can without stopping.

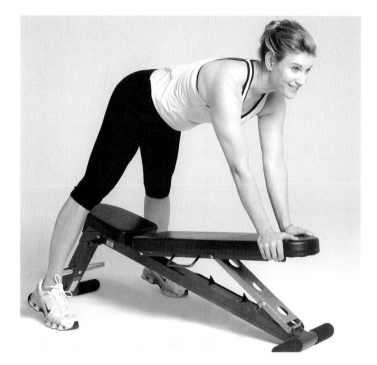

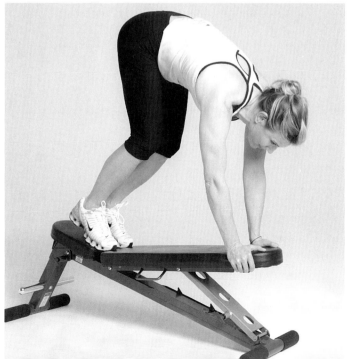

2. Reverse Lunge with Medicine Ball

Strengthens front thighs, buttocks, and rear thighs.

Stand tall, holding a medicine ball with both hands. Step backward with your right foot and bend both knees into a lunge. Your left knee should be directly over your left ankle, your right heel lifted. Touch the ball on the floor by the outside of your left foot. Straighten your legs, pushing off your back foot to return to the starting position. This equals one rep. Do 10 reps, then switch legs and repeat.

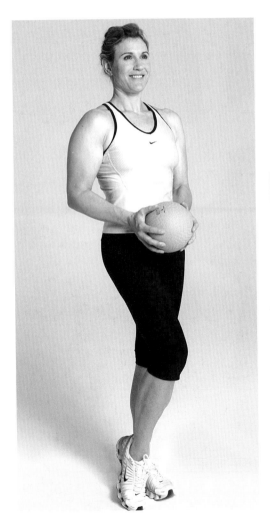
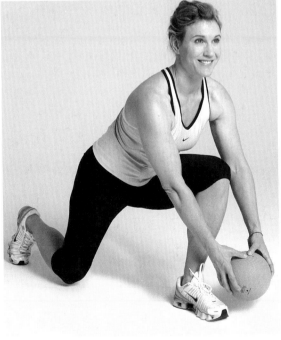

3. Shoulder Shaper

Strengthens shoulders.

Hold a dumbbell in each hand, using an overhand grip. Sit on the edge of a bench (you can use a chair, if you don't have a bench) and hold the weights above your shoulders. Exhale as you press the dumbbells straight up. Pause, then slowly return to the starting position. This equals one rep. Do 2 sets of 12 reps. *Recommended weight range: 5 to 15 pounds.*

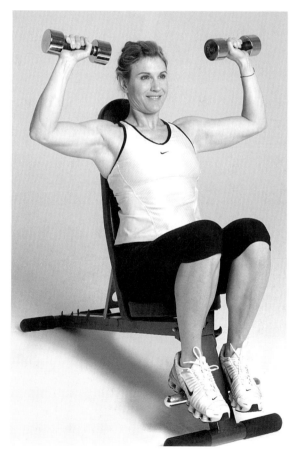
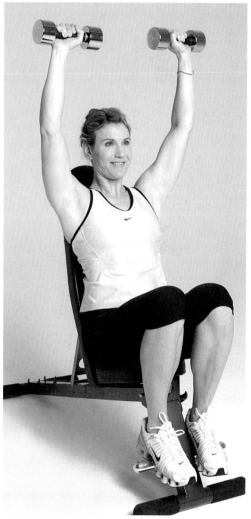

4. Squat-to-Knee Strike

Stand with your feet hip width apart and hands on your hips. Bend your knees and lower your-self into a squat position; at the same time, raise your arms straight out in front of you, level with your shoulders. Slowly straighten your legs to a standing position, shifting your weight onto your left leg as you bring the right toe to the inside of your left knee. Return your hands to your hips. This equals one rep. Hold, then repeat. After 8 reps, switch legs and repeat. Do 2 sets of 8 reps on each side.

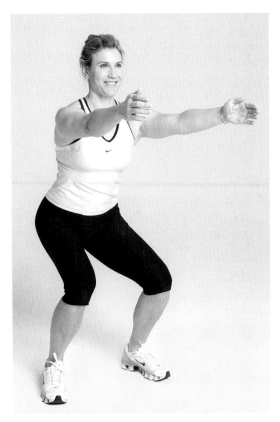 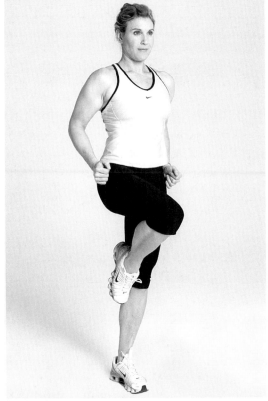

5. Side Lunge with Upright Row

Hold a dumbbell in each hand, arms hanging down in front of you, palms facing in. Take a big step to the right with your right foot and bend your right knee into a side lunge; at the same time, lift your elbows until they're level with your shoulders. Lower your arms and step back into the starting position. This equals one rep. Do 10 reps with your right leg, then switch legs and repeat. *Recommended weight range: 5 to 10 pounds.*

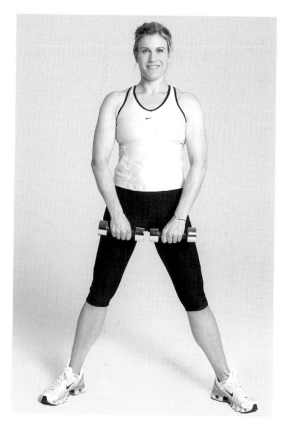
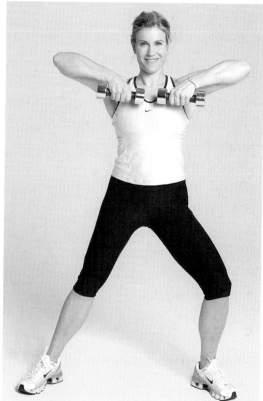

6. Straight-Arm Press Back

Strengthens back, rear shoulders, and rear arms.

Attach a resistance tube with a handle to a sturdy pole (or use the doorjamb apparatus that comes with some resistance tubes). Hold the handle in your right hand, then step back slightly more than arm's length away. Keeping your back straight, bend forward at your hips until your torso is parallel to the floor. Extend your right arm in front of you, palm facing down, abs pulled in. Press your right arm down and behind you until it's even with your back, palm facing up. Hold, then slowly return to the starting position. This equals one rep. After 12 reps, switch arms and repeat. Do 2 sets of 12 reps with each arm.

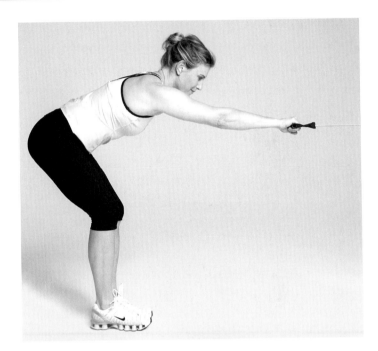

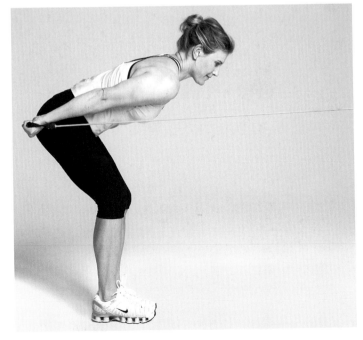

7. Straight-Leg Dead Lift

Strengthens buttocks and rear thighs.

Holding a dumbbell in each hand with an overhand grip, stand with your feet together, abs pulled in. Keeping your back straight and knees slightly bent, bend forward at your hips and lower your torso toward the floor until you feel a stretch in your hamstrings, with your arms hanging straight down. Pause, then contract your buttocks and hamstrings as you slowly return to the starting position. This equals one rep. Do 2 sets of 10 reps. *Recommended weight range: 5 to 15 pounds.*

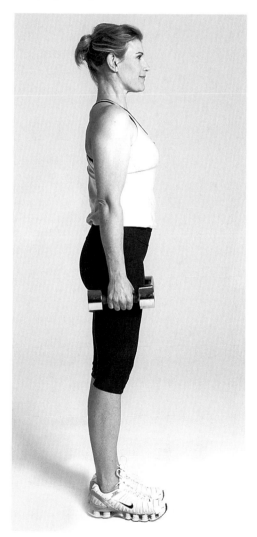

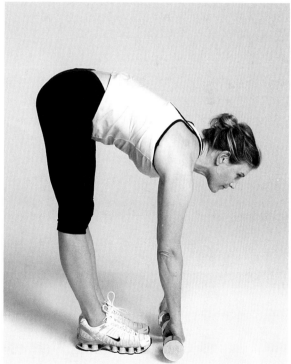

8. Plank Push-Up Rotation

Strengthens chest, back of upper arms, front shoulders, lower body, and core.

To modify this exercise, do it in a bent-knee push-up position instead of a plank. **Kneel on all fours with your knees directly below your hips and with your hands in line with your shoulders. Your elbows should be slightly bent, fingers spread apart, abs pulled in. Extend your legs out behind you, so your body forms a straight line from your head to your heels. This is the plank position. Bend your arms and lower your chest to the floor, until your elbows are level with your shoulders. Exhale as you straighten your arms to return to the plank position. Next, rotate your body to the right, so you're balanced on your right hand and the outside edge of your right foot, and extend your left arm to the ceiling. Hold, then return to the plank position. Repeat, rotating to the left. Return to the plank position. This equals one rep. Do 4–8 reps.**

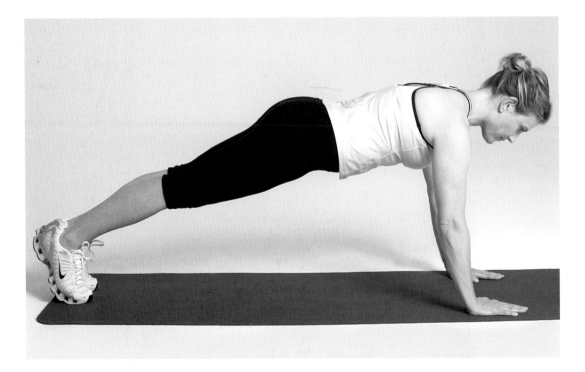

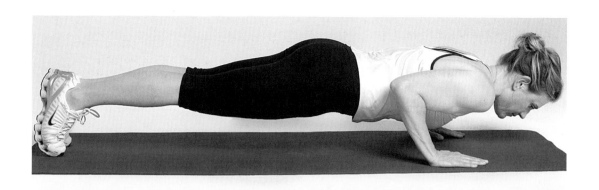

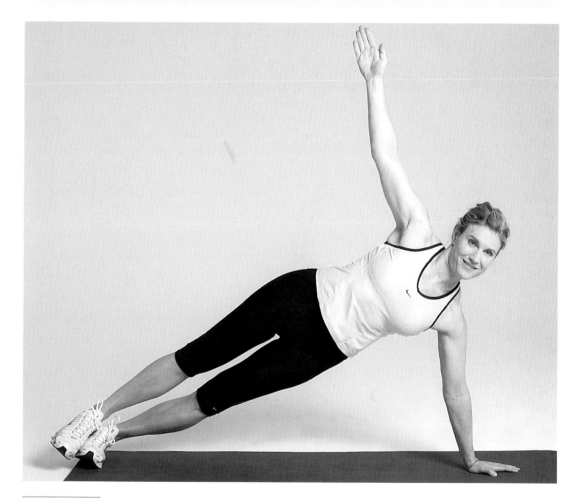

Cool down. Finish with the Stretch and Unwind routine on page 119.

Tuesday/Day Two:
Cardio (Core Walk) and Ab Workout

Tuesday Core Walk

Total distance: 3 miles

Total workout time: 39 minutes

Your walking workout. Your first cardio workout of the week consists of a simple 3-mile walk.

Week 1: If you're walking outdoors, you'll need to map out a 3-mile walking route, if you haven't already done so. (See page 59 for details.) When you're ready to walk, grab your sports watch or stopwatch. Your goal is to walk the 3 miles as fast as you can. Time yourself and see how long it takes. This will be your base time.

Week 2 and after: Continue trying to improve your time. Your ultimate goal is to walk the 3 miles at a 13-minutes-per-mile pace (or about 4.6 miles per hour, if you're using a treadmill). This should take 39 minutes.

Once you've reached this goal, you can keep increasing your pace, add more miles, or incorporate hills (find a hilly place to walk or crank up the incline on your treadmill). Or you can boost the intensity by

wearing a weighted vest. I like the X2 vest (800-697-5658; www.x2vest
.com) because it allows you to add weight in 1-pound increments.

On all your walks, be sure to use the proper walking technique: Stand
tall with your chest and chin lifted and your abs pulled in. Your shoulders should be back and relaxed, not hunched. Swing your arms comfortably, in a natural rhythm with your stride.

As soon as you finish walking, grab your large exercise ball and an
exercise mat and do the following ab routine.

Abs

1. Abdominal Crunch on the Ball

Strengthens core; front thighs and buttocks work as stabilizers.

Sit on a large exercise ball, then tuck your pelvis, lean back, and walk your feet away from the ball until your back is supported on the ball and the bottom of your shoulder blades are barely touching the ball. Cradle your head in your hands, elbows wide, and focus up at the ceiling. Exhale as you curl your upper body up as far as you can, pulling your belly button toward your spine. Slowly return to the starting position. This equals one rep. Try to not let the ball move while you do this exercise. Do 2 sets of 20 reps.

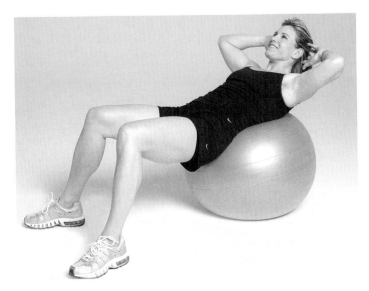

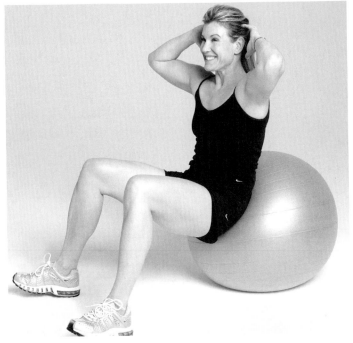

2. Torso Rotation with Dumbbell

Strengthens core, with an emphasis on the obliques (sides of the waist); front thighs and buttocks work as stabilizers.

Start by doing this exercise without a dumbbell. Once you're comfortable with the move, add a 3- or 5-pound weight. Sit on a large exercise ball, holding a dumbbell by its ends. Lean back and walk your feet forward until you're in a bridge position, with your hips elevated; your head, neck, and upper back should be supported on the ball. Extend your arms straight up, so you're holding the dumbbell overhead. Keeping your arms straight, rotate your torso and arms to the right, lifting your left shoulder up off the ball. Return back to the center, then rotate to the left. Rotate back to the center. This equals one rep. Do 20 reps. *Recommended weight range: 3 to 5 pounds.*

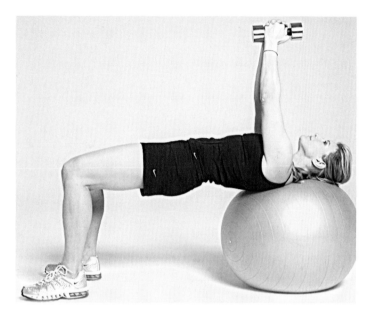

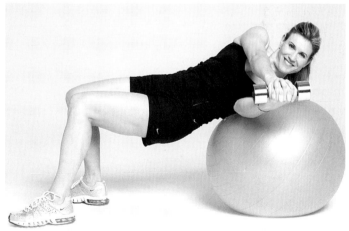

3. Pike on the Ball

If this exercise is too challenging, modify it by bringing your knees in toward your chest rather than lifting your hips. Lie on top of a large exercise ball with your hands on the floor in front of you and your abs pulled in. Walk your hands forward until your lower legs rest on the center of the ball, arms straight, wrists in line with your shoulders. Use your core muscles to lift your hips into a pike position or inverted V. As you do this, the ball should roll down along your shins. Slowly return to the starting position, with your thighs on top of the ball. This equals one rep. Do 2 sets of 4–6 reps.

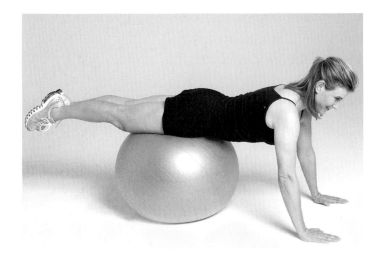

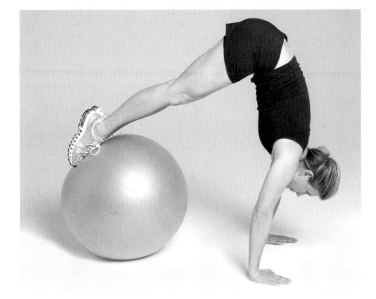

4. Ab Roller

Kneel in front of a large exercise ball. Place your hands on top of the ball, with your arms straight. Tighten your abs and curl your upper body forward as you roll the ball away from you as far as you can. Hold, then roll back to the starting position. This equals one rep. Do 2 sets of 5–8 reps.

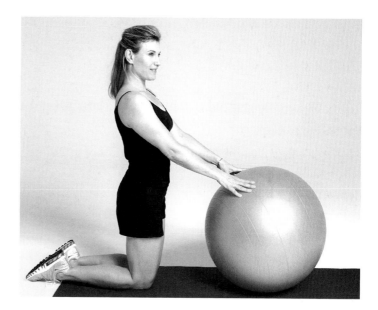

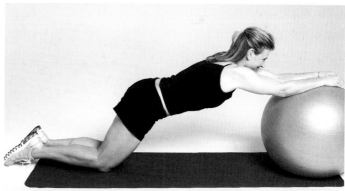

5. Windshield Wiper

Strengthens core, with an emphasis on the obliques (sides of your waist).

Lie on your back with a large exercise ball between your feet and your arms out to the sides. Squeeze the ball between your feet and lift your legs toward the ceiling, until they're at a 90-degree angle. Keeping your right shoulder against the floor, lower your legs to your left. Go as far as you can without letting the ball touch the floor. Use your core muscles to pull the ball back up to the starting position, then repeat to the other side. This equals one rep. Do 2 sets of 8 reps.

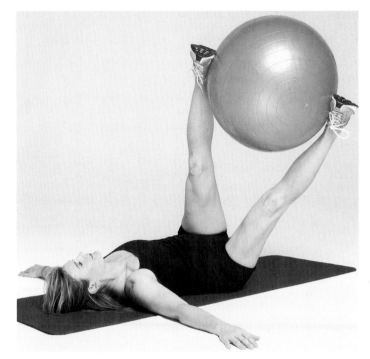

Cool down. After your last ab exercise, continue lying on your back with your legs resting on the ball. Close your eyes and relax for a minute. Then do 10 to 20 Kegels. Finish with the Stretch and Unwind routine on page 119.

Wednesday/Day Three:
Strength Workout

Warm up. Start with 5 minutes of low-intensity cardio, such as walking or marching in place.

Your strength workout. Do the following exercises in the order listed. Rest 30 to 60 seconds between sets.

1. Lunge Kick

Strengthens front thighs, rear thighs, and buttocks.

Stand tall with your feet hip width apart and your abs pulled in, arms at your sides with dumbbells in each hand. Step backward with your right foot and bend both knees into a lunge. Your left knee should be directly over your left ankle, your right heel lifted. As you come back, follow the right leg through with a high kick with the foot flexed. At the same time, bend your elbows and lift your hands toward your shoulders in a bicep curl motion. Step the right leg back again and lower your arms. This equals one rep. Do 10 reps, then switch legs and repeat. Do 2 sets of 10 reps with each leg. *Recommended weight range: 3 to 8 pounds.*

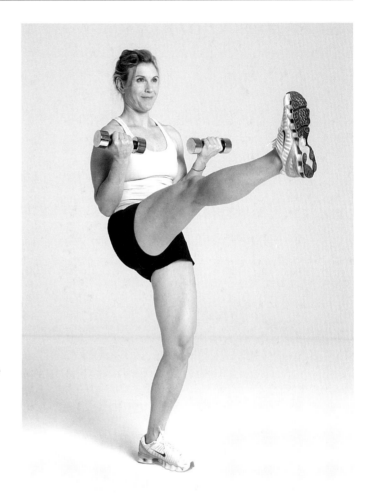

2. Bridge Chest Press on the Ball

Strengthens chest, core, front thighs, and buttocks.

Lie on a large exercise ball with your shoulders supported, your knees bent at a 90-degree angle, your feet shoulder width apart, and your abs pulled in tight. Keep your hips lifted so your body is in a straight line from head to knees. Hold a dumbbell in each hand, with your palms facing inward. Slowly lower the dumbbells down toward your armpits. Hold for a few seconds, then press back up to the starting position. This equals one rep. Do 2 sets of 12 reps. *Recommended weight range: 5 to 15 pounds.*

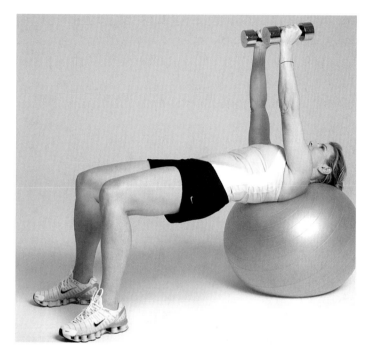

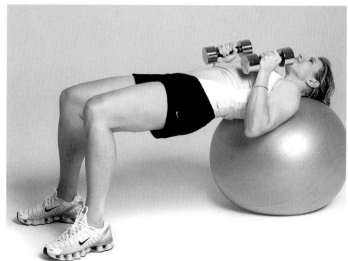

3. Cross-Legged Squat

Strengthens front thighs, buttocks, and rear thighs.

Stand on your right leg with your right knee slightly bent. Cross your left leg over your right leg, just above your knee, as if you're sitting with your legs crossed. Extend your arms out in front of you for balance. Bend your right knee until your left foot touches the floor. Keep your back straight and tilt your upper body slightly forward. As you lower yourself, you will feel the outside of your right thigh contract. As you return to the starting position, you will feel it in the hamstring muscles on the back of your right thigh. This equals one rep. Do 2 sets of 10 reps on each side.

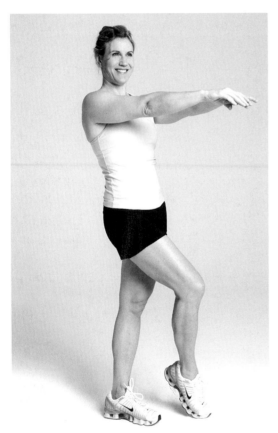 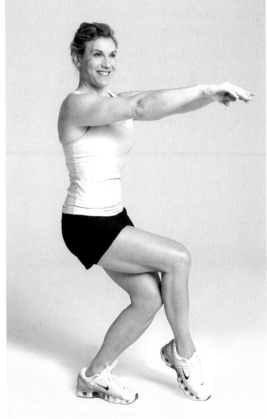

4. Side Leg Lifts on the Ball

Strengthens outer thighs and core.

Kneel on the floor with a large exercise ball next to your left side. Lean into the ball and contour the space between your rib cage and pelvis into the ball. Place your hands behind your head. If you aren't comfortable, you can place one hand on the ball. Straighten your right leg and lift it up to hip level. Don't move your hips or pelvis away from the ball. Lower your leg back to the floor. This equals one rep. Do 2 sets of 10 reps on each side.

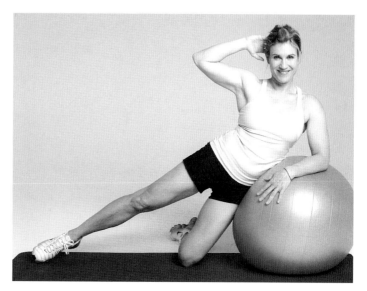

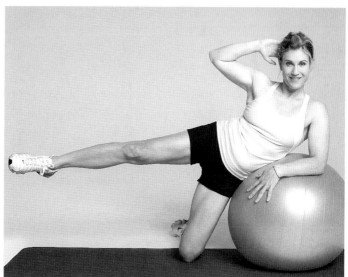

5. Reverse Fly on the Ball

Strengthens rear shoulders, back, and core.

Do this exercise without dumb-bells until you feel stable and balanced. Start by using 3-pound weights, and gradually work up to 8 pounds in each hand. Lie on a large exercise ball so your belly is on the center and your legs are extended straight back with your toes on the floor. Your body should form a straight line from your head to your heels. Grasp a dumbbell in each hand. Squeeze your shoulder blades together and pull your arms into a wide arc, keeping your elbows slightly bent. Hold, then slowly lower your arms. This equals one rep. Do 2 sets of 10 reps. *Recommended weight range: 3 to 8 pounds.*

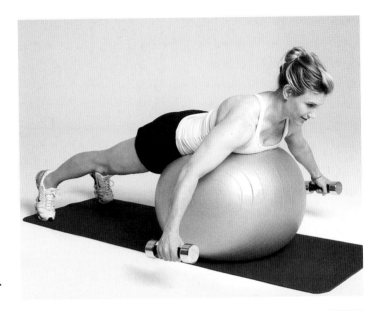

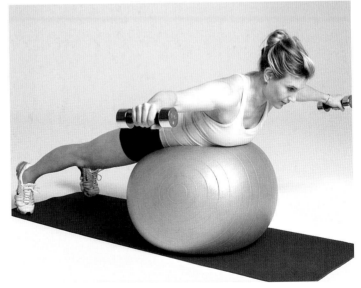

6. One-Arm Triceps Push-Up

Strengthens back of arms.

Lie on your right side with your left palm flat on the floor in front of your shoulder, elbow bent. Wrap your right arm around your waist. Using your left arm, push your torso up until the arm is straight. Then lower your upper body until your shoulder is about an inch from the floor. This equals one rep. Be sure to keep your hips and feet planted on the floor. Keep your shoulders down and relaxed; don't hunch them. Do 8–10 reps, then switch sides and repeat. Do 2 sets of 8–10 reps with each arm.

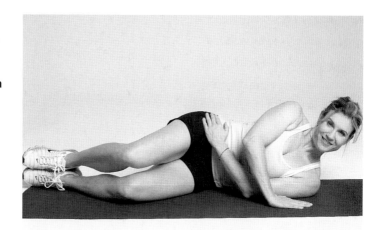

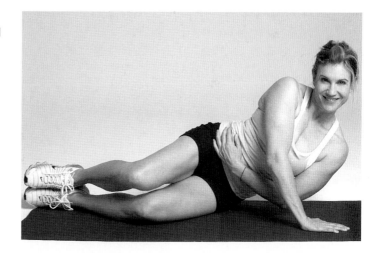

7. One-Legged Push-Up

Strengthens chest, shoulders, and back of arms.

To modify this exercise, keep the toe of your extended leg on the floor. Come into a push-up position with your knees bent on the floor, your hands slightly wider than shoulder width apart and underneath your shoulders, and your elbows slightly bent. Extend your right leg behind you to form a straight line from your heel to your head. Bend your arms until your elbows are level with your shoulders. Exhale as you straighten your arms to return to the starting position. This equals one rep. Do 3 sets of 8–10 reps.

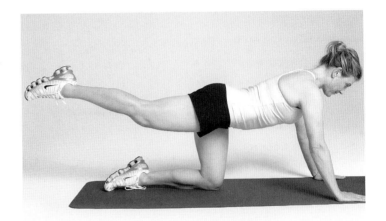

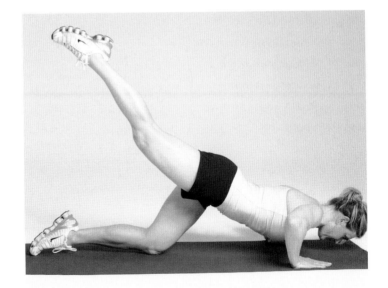

8. Bridge Leg Curl

Strengthens rear thighs and buttocks.

Lie on your back with your arms relaxed at your side. Place your feet on a large exercise ball so that the ball rests under your lower legs and your legs are extended straight. Lift your pelvis off the floor so your body forms a straight line from your shoulders to your feet. Keeping your pelvis lifted, bend your knees and roll the ball in toward your buttocks with your feet. Slowly straighten your legs and roll the ball back to the starting position. This equals one rep. Don't arch your back. Do 2 sets of 25 reps. (You may have to work up to 25 reps.)

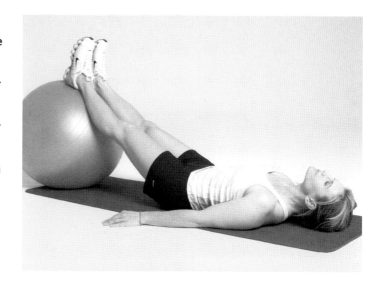

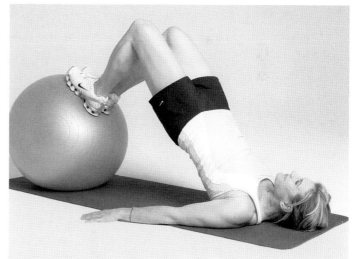

Cool down. Finish with the Stretch and Unwind routine on page 119.

Thursday/Day Four:
Cardio (Walk Circuit) and Ab Workout

Thursday Walk Circuit

Total distance: 3 miles

Total workout time: 1 hour

Your walking workout. Today, you'll be doing another 3-mile walk. But this time you'll add in quick cardio blasts to really get your heart pumping. Here's how: Start walking at a brisk pace. At the end of each mile, stop and do the four moves described next. These moves are fun and easy to do. You'll really feel your heart rate soar and your muscles wake up. Do each move 20 times. As soon as you're finished, start walking again! Note: If your walking route isn't conducive to performing these moves at each mile marker, save them until the end and do them inside your home.

1. Running Man Hands Down

Kneel on all fours, then extend your legs behind you in a straight-leg push-up or plank position. Keeping your hands on the ground, bend your right knee and bring it into your chest. Extend it back to the starting position, then bring your left knee into your chest. Continue alternating legs as if you're running. Do 20 reps with each leg. If this is too hard on your wrists, do the move standing, with your hands firmly placed on a low wall or bench.

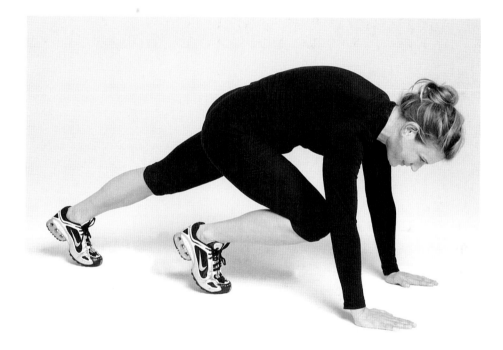

2. Exploding Squat Jumps

Stand with your feet together and your knees slightly bent. Bend both knees and lower your hips down into a squat. Keeping your feet together, straighten your legs and jump up and to the right, getting as high off the ground as you can. Land softly with your knees slightly bent and immediately lower yourself into another squat, then jump back to the other side. Back and forth equals one rep. Do 20 reps.

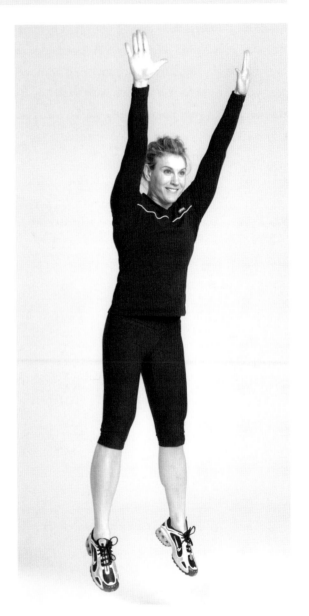

3. Full-Out Plank Jacks

Kneel on all fours and extend your legs into a straight-leg push-up position. Separate your feet wider than your shoulders. Your hands should be directly under your shoulders, abs pulled in tight to protect your back. Keep your torso straight; don't sag at your hips. Without moving your hands or your torso, jump your feet together, then back apart again. This equals one rep. Do 20 reps total.

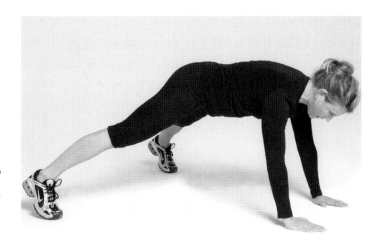

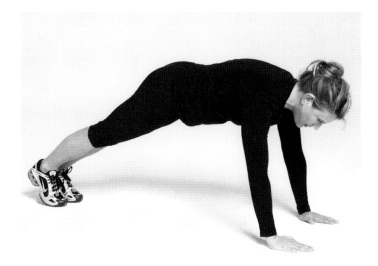

4. Squat Kick

Stand with your feet shoulder width apart. Bend your knees and lower your hips into a squat. Straighten your legs to return to the starting position, then kick one leg up as high as you can in front of you. Keep your abs pulled in tight. The kick should be quick but very controlled. Immediately lower your leg and repeat with the opposite leg. Both legs equals one rep. Do 20 reps.

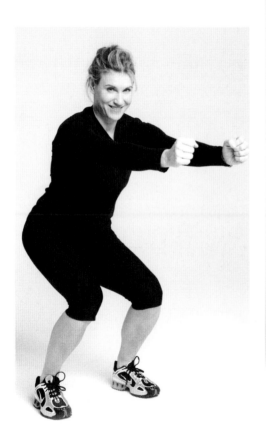
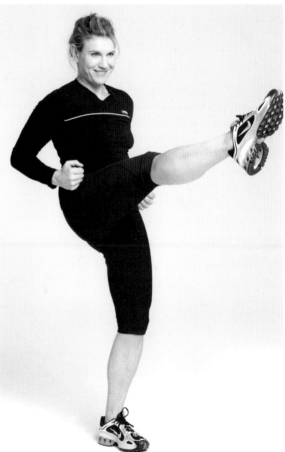

After the last cardio blast, walk for a few minutes to let your heart rate return to normal, then move right to your ab routine.

Abs

1. Plank Hold

Kneel on all fours, then bend your arms and place your elbows on the floor directly under your shoulders. Your forearms should point straight ahead, palms facing down. Extend your legs out behind you, so you're supported on your forearms and toes. Pull your abs in tight, as if you're wearing a corset. Your body should form a straight line from your head to your feet. Press your shoulders back and down toward your waistline. Hold this position for a count of 60. If you cannot make it to 60, lower yourself down and rest, then try it again. To make this move even more challenging, lift one leg off the ground and hold for 30 seconds, then switch legs and repeat.

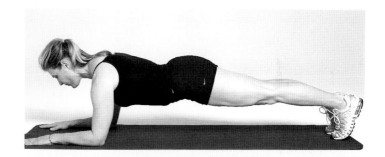

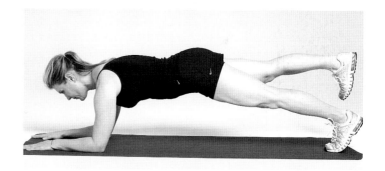

2. Straight-Arm Side Bridge

Lie on your right hip with the outer side of your right leg flat on the floor and your upper body propped up on your right arm. Pushing against the floor with your right arm, raise your hips and legs off the floor. Extend your left arm straight up and form a T with your body. Hold for a moment, then return to the floor. This equals one rep. Do 5 reps on each side.

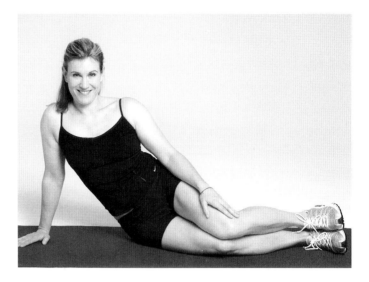

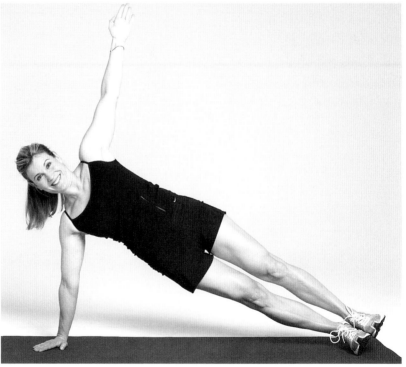

3. Toe Touch

Lie on your back with a medium-sized ball between your feet. (If the medicine ball is too heavy, you can use any other type of ball, such as a dodgeball, soccer ball, basketball, or small beach ball.) Lift your legs and arms straight up in the air as high as you can. Exhale and use your abs to curl up, lifting your shoulders off the ground. Try to touch the ball with your fingertips. Pause, then lower yourself and return to the starting position. This equals one rep. Do 2 sets of 15 reps.

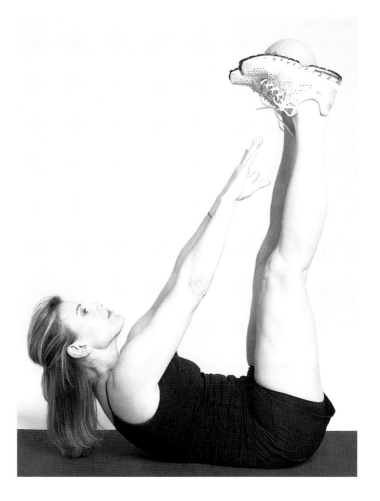

4. Side Jackknife

Lie on your right side with your legs straight. Support your upper body on your right elbow and forearm. Your elbow should be directly under your shoulder, your forearm pointing in front of you. Rest your left hand behind your head by your left ear. Point your elbow toward your feet. Lift your legs toward your torso while keeping your torso still. Pause to feel the contraction on the right side of the waist. Slowly lower your legs. This equals one rep. After 10 reps, switch sides and repeat. Do 2 sets of 10 reps on each side.

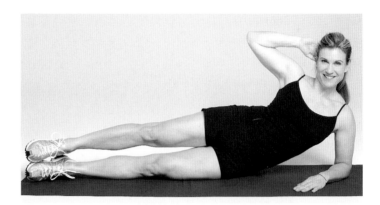

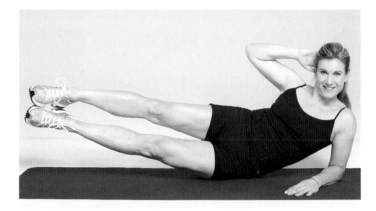

5. Medicine Ball Torso Twist

Kneel on the floor, holding a medicine ball in front of you. Sit back on your heels. Twist to the right and set the ball down directly behind you. Twist to the left, pick up the ball, and bring it back around to your right again. Set the ball down and repeat the circle. Once around equals one rep. Do 8 reps, then switch directions and repeat.

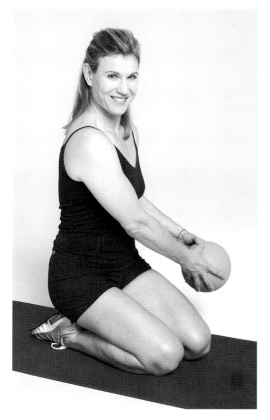
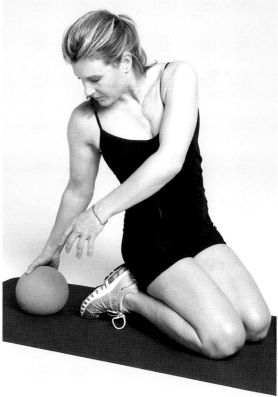

Friday/Day Five:
Strength Workout

Warm up. Start with 5 minutes of low-intensity cardio, such as walking or marching in place.

Your strength workout. Do the following exercises in the order listed. Rest 30 to 60 seconds between sets.

1. Side Lunge Balance

Strengthens front thighs, buttocks, and core.

Stand with your feet hip width apart. Take a big step to the right with your right foot. Bend your right knee until your right thigh is parallel to the floor. Push off your right foot and pull your right knee up until it is level with your hip. Hold for 2 to 3 counts. Slowly lower yourself to the starting position. This equals one rep. Do 8 reps, rest for 30 seconds, then switch legs and repeat. Do 2 sets of 8 reps with each leg.

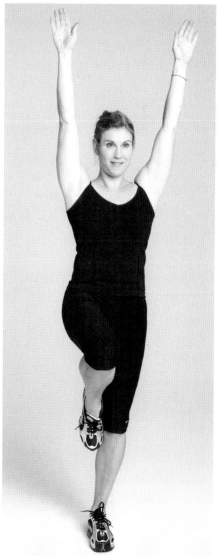

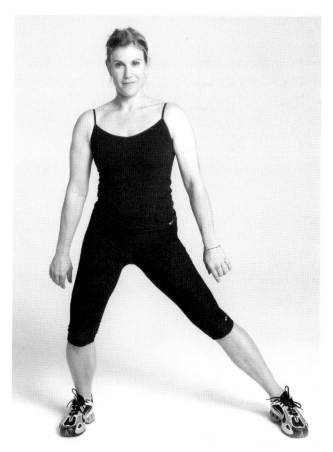

2. Triceps Kickback

Grasp a dumbbell in your right hand, then stand with your feet together. Keeping your back straight, hinge forward at your hips, bending your knees slightly. Bend your right arm at a 90-degree angle, keeping your elbow in close to your side. Squeeze the back of your arm as you slowly extend your arm behind you, keeping your elbow close to your side. Although this exercise implies a quick movement, don't use momentum. Slowly return to the starting position. This equals one rep. Do 2 sets of 12 reps on each arm. *Recommended weight range: 5 to 10 pounds.*

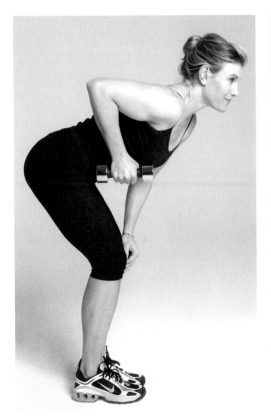 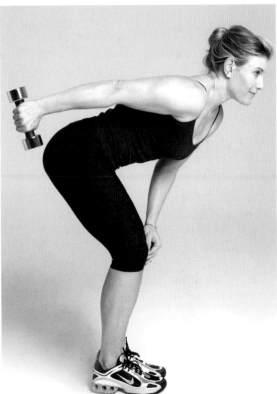

3. Reverse Lunge Torso Rotation

Strengthens front thighs, rear thighs, buttocks, and core.

Stand with your feet together. Hold a dumbbell with both hands just in front of your thighs. Raise the weight straight out in front of you, then step backward with your right foot and bend both knees into a lunge. Your left knee should be directly over your left ankle, your right heel lifted. Keep your abs tight and rotate your torso and the dumbbell toward your right leg. Hold for a moment, then rotate back, simultaneously bringing your right leg back to the starting position. Repeat the exercise, lunging with your left leg. This equals one rep. Do 10 reps. *Recommended weight range: 5 to 15 pounds.*

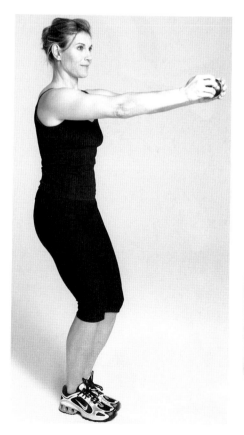 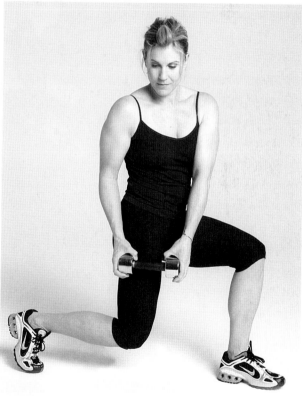

4. Seated Biceps Curl

Hold a dumbbell in your right hand with an underhand grip and sit on a bench. (If you don't have a bench, you can use a large exercise ball or a sturdy chair.) Lean forward slightly and let the weight hang straight down, with your arm fully extended and the back of your upper arm resting against the inside of your thigh. Rest the other arm on your other thigh. Keeping your wrist straight, bend your elbow to curl the weight up toward your shoulder without moving your upper arm or torso. Slowly return to the starting position. This equals one rep. Do 10 reps, then switch arms and repeat. Do 3 sets of 10 reps with each arm. *Recommended weight range: 5 to 15 pounds.*

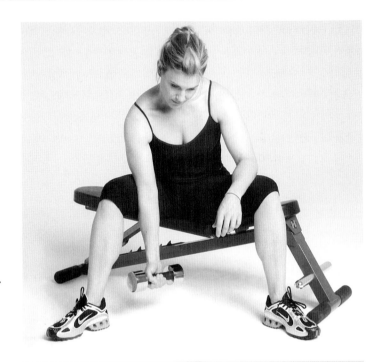

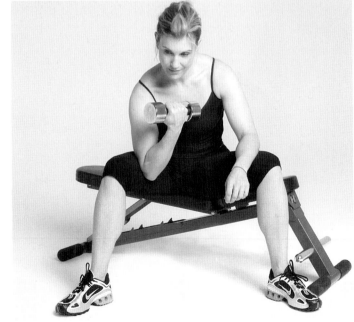

5. Front Raise Stationary Lunge

Stand with your feet together and one end of a resistance band under your right foot. Hold the other end of the band and a dumbbell in your left hand. Step backward with your left foot into a lunge. Your right knee should be directly over your right ankle, right knee slightly bent, left heel lifted. Straighten your legs as you extend your left arm (holding the weight and band) straight out in front of you at shoulder level. Pause, then lower your left arm back to your side as you bend your knees back into the lunge position. This equals one rep. Do 8 reps, then switch sides and repeat. Do 2 sets of 8 reps on each side. *Recommended weight range: 3 to 8 pounds.*

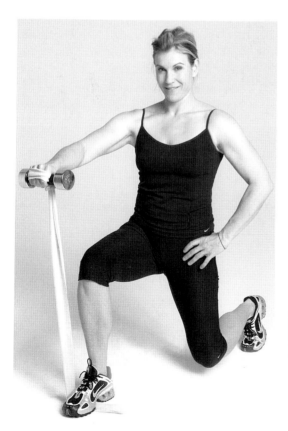
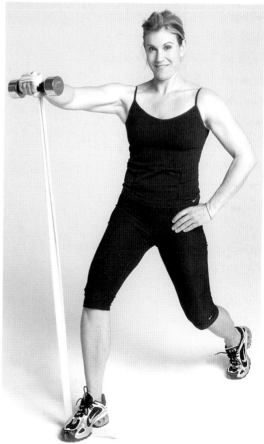

6. Side-Lying Scissors

Strengthens front thighs, rear thighs, buttocks, hip flexors, and core.

*To make this move even more challenging, place both hands behind your head as you do
the scissors.* Lie on your right side with your head supported on your right arm. Extend your

legs and keep your body in a
straight line with your hips
stacked, legs together, and
toes pointed. Place your left
hand in front of you for balance. Lift your legs a few
inches off the floor. Bring your
right leg forward and your left
leg back without shifting your
hips. This equals one rep. Inhale and exhale throughout
the exercise as you scissor your
legs forward and back. Do
10 reps, then repeat the move
lying on your left side.

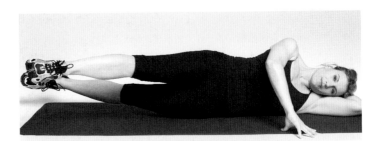

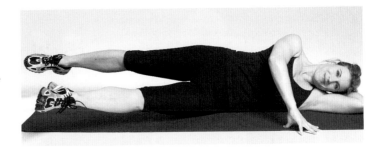

7. Ball Extension

For an even bigger challenge, do this move with your palms facing up, so you can't press down with your arms. Lie on the floor with a large exercise ball between your feet, arms extended to the sides, palms facing down. Lift your knees so they're bent over your hips. Press your lower back into the floor and tighten your abs. Exhale as you straighten your legs and lift the ball toward the ceiling, keeping your knees over your hips. Slowly lower yourself back to the starting position. This equals one rep. Do 2 sets of 8–10 reps.

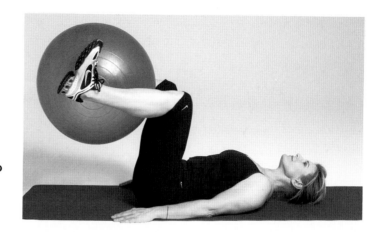

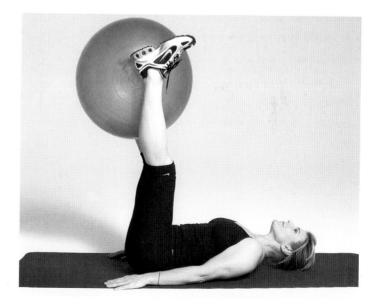

8. Balance Push-Up

Strengthens triceps (back of arms), shoulders, and chest.

To modify this exercise, do a basic bent-knee push-up, with your hands slightly wider than shoulder width apart and underneath your shoulders, and both knees on the floor. Start in a bent-knee push-up position, then extend your right leg behind you and your right arm out to the side and slightly behind your body at shoulder level. Balancing on your left knee and left palm, lower your chest toward the floor. Slowly return to the starting position. This equals one rep. Do 8–10 reps, then switch sides and repeat.

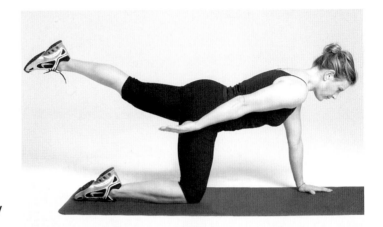

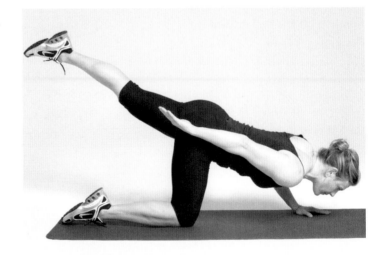

Saturday/Day Six:
Cardio (Walk/Run Intervals) and Ab Workout

Total distance: 3 miles

Total workout time: 40 minutes

Your walking workout. For your third cardio session, you'll be incorporating some short running intervals into your 3-mile walk. This is a great way to boost your intensity and incinerate calories. Plus it will make the time fly by!

Be sure you have your stopwatch or sports watch set on chrono mode (the timer). In the workout, you'll be alternating intervals of brisk walking and fast running. (If you're using a treadmill, your walking pace should be about 4 to 4.5 miles per hour; your running pace should be about 6 to 8 miles per hour. Each walking interval will last 3 to 5 minutes. The running intervals will range from 30 seconds to 2 minutes.

Copy the following chart and carry it in your pocket or tape it onto your treadmill. Or better yet, memorize the routine. Each week, try to improve your time and increase the length of your sprints. If you're just getting back into shape and a full-out sprint is too challenging for you, just pick up the pace as much as you can. You can start with brisk walking, then build up to jogging as your fitness level improves. Try to go a little faster each time, working toward the goal of a 6- to 8-miles-per-hour running pace.

Walk/run intervals

>5-minute walk
>
>:30 second sprint
>
>5-minute walk
>
>1:00 minute sprint
>
>5-minute walk
>
>1:30 minute sprint
>
>3-minute walk
>
>2:00 minute sprint
>
>3-minute walk
>
>1:30 minute sprint
>
>3-minute walk
>
>1:00 minute sprint
>
>5-minute walk
>
>:30 second sprint

To cool down, walk slowly until your heart rate returns to normal. Then start on your ab routine.

Abs

This workout focuses on your obliques, or the abdominal muscles that run along the sides of your waist.

1. Waist Whittler

Strengthens core, with an emphasis on the obliques (sides of the waist).

Lie on your right side with your body supported on your right forearm and elbow, and your knees bent at a 90-degree angle and in line with your body, with your feet behind you. Lift your hips so your body forms a straight line from head to knees. Hold for 5 counts. Return to the floor. This equals one rep. Do 5–8 reps, then switch sides and repeat.

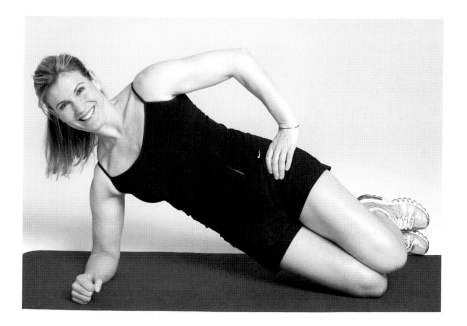

2. Reverse Ab Thrust

Strengthens core, with an emphasis on the obliques (sides of the waist).

Lie on your back on a bench with your legs bent and your feet resting lightly on the bench. Reach up behind you and hold the bench behind your head. Engage your abs and pull your belly button toward your spine. Lift and thrust your hips off the bench as high as you can, pushing your feet straight up. Slowly lower your hips to the starting position. This equals one rep. Start with 15 reps and gradually build up to 25 reps.

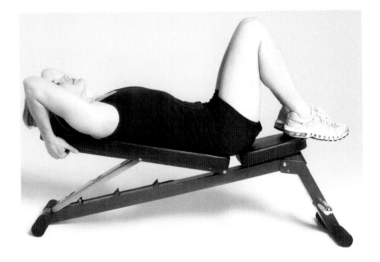

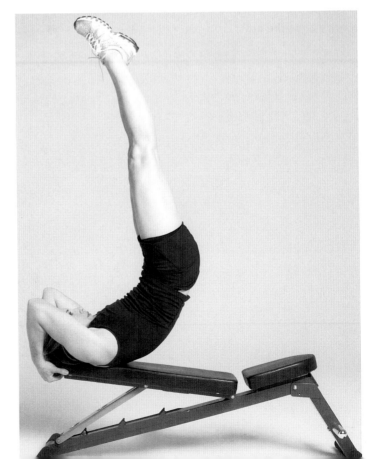

3. Dumbbell Cross Reach

Strengthens core, with an emphasis on the obliques (sides of the waist).

If 5-pound dumbbells are too heavy, start with 3 pounds in each hand and switch to heavier weights once you're stronger. Holding a dumbbell in each hand, lie on your back with your legs straight up in the air and rest the weights near your shoulders. Exhale as you use your abs to lift your shoulders off the ground. Reach your right hand (with the dumbbell) toward your left foot, then return to the starting position and lower your shoulders back down to the floor. Repeat the move, reaching your left arm toward your right foot. This equals one rep. To make it more challenging, keep your shoulders hovering off the ground instead of lowering them to the floor between reaches. If you feel tension in your neck, relax and place your tongue against the roof of your mouth. Do 2 sets of 8 reps. *Recommended weight range: 3 to 5 pounds.*

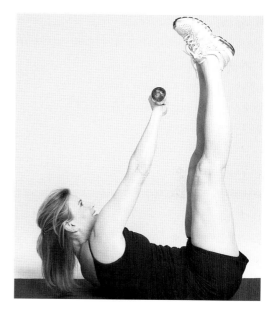

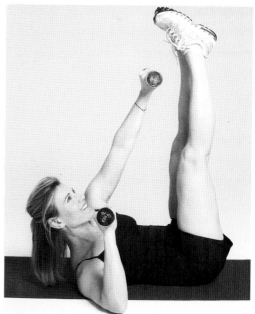

4. Side Plank Rotation

Strengthens core, with an emphasis on the obliques (sides of the waist).

To modify this exercise, try scissoring your legs (so one is in front of the other) instead of keeping them stacked. Place a dumbbell on the floor. Get into a right-side plank position: Lie on your right side with your body supported on your forearm and elbow, legs straight, hips and feet stacked. Your hips should be raised slightly off the floor so your body forms a straight line from head to toe. Be sure your right shoulder is directly over your elbow. Keeping your abs engaged and hips lifted, grasp the dumbbell with your left hand and extend your arm straight up. Then slowly lower the weight down, rotating your torso toward the floor until you feel your obliques contract. The weight should be slightly underneath you. This equals one rep. Do 5–10 reps, then switch sides and repeat. *Recommended weight range: 3 to 5 pounds.*

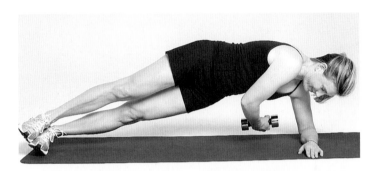

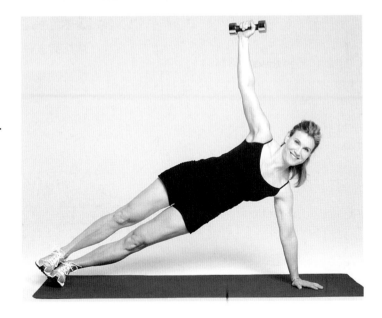

5. Twist and Turn

Strengthens core, with an emphasis on the obliques (sides of the waist).

Lie face up on the floor, holding a medicine ball in both hands, with your knees bent and your feet flat on the floor. Tighten your abs and extend your arms straight up over your chest. Keeping your abs pulled in, rotate your upper body to the right, reaching your arms to the side and lowering the ball toward the floor; simultaneously rotate your lower body to the left, lowering your knees toward the floor. Don't let your knees or the ball touch the floor. Exhale as you use your abs to lift your arms and legs to the starting position. Pause, then repeat, lowering your arms to the left side and knees to the right. Exhale as you return to the starting position. This equals one rep. Do 8 reps. Be sure to exhale every time you return to center.

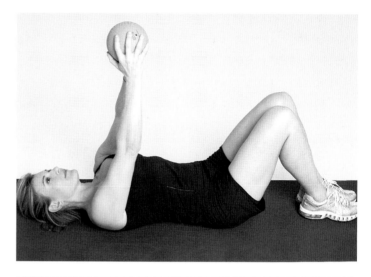

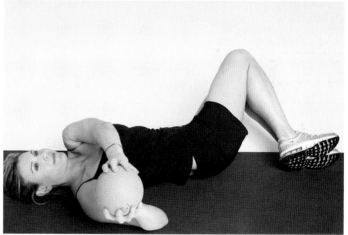

Cool down. Finish with the Stretch and Unwind routine on page 119.

Sunday/Day Seven:
"Free" Day

This is your day off, so how you spend it is up to you. But I urge you to do at least one good thing for your body—whether it's relaxing in a warm bath, getting a massage, or doing something fun and active. I love to spend my Sundays walking around a flea market, playing basketball with my kids, bike riding with my husband, or going for a long hike with my dogs.

Also, before the day is over, take a moment to flip through your fitness journal and reflect on how much you've accomplished. Give yourself a pat on the back for all your hard work. Think about how good you look. Think about how great you feel. Sit down and plan your workouts for the coming week. Keep up the excellent work . . . even if you don't see any visible changes yet, you're benefiting your body in countless ways!

Stretch and Unwind

Ahhhh . . . stretching. It feels so good and it's so incredibly good for our bodies. Our muscles are like rubber bands and are incredibly resilient. But the less we use them, the tighter they get. By stretching regularly, we can keep them limber and increase our range of motion so we move better and avoid injuries. We can also combat everyday aches and pains caused by hours spent sitting in our cars, in front of computers, and on the couch. Still, despite all the known benefits, most of us still neglect to do it. I'll admit that I'm as guilty as the next person. Whenever I'm in a hurry, my post-workout stretches are the first thing to go. But with each passing year, I become more aware of what a mistake that is. When I don't stretch, my muscles don't recover as quickly, and I'm more likely to feel stiff and sore the next day. The bottom line: Now that we're getting older, we can't afford to overlook stretching anymore.

The following stretching routine consists of eight feel-good moves. Do the entire sequence at the end of each daily workout, or whenever you're feeling stiff or stressed out. Memorize the moves and try to flow smoothly from one to the next. Inhale deeply through your nose and exhale through your mouth as you hold each stretch. Focus on lengthening your muscles. Take this time to slow down, focus inward, and feel your breath flowing through your body. Enjoy!

1. Body Curve

Sit on the floor with your knees bent, your feet flat on the floor, and your hands clasping your knees. Round your back and pull your belly button in toward your spine. Inhale through your nose, keeping your chin near your chest. As you exhale, slowly rock forward and back a few times. Take 5 deep breaths. After the last breath, slowly lower yourself onto your back and lie down.

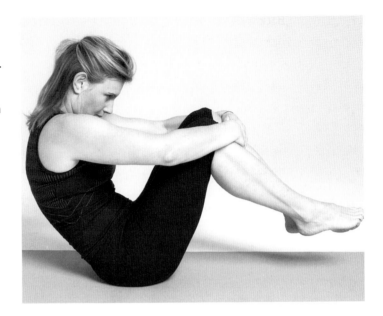

2. Hamstring Stretch

Lying on your back with your legs extended straight in front of you, bend your right knee into your chest. Interlace your fingers behind the back of your right thigh and gently pull your leg in toward you until you feel a gentle tension. Extend your right leg straight up in the air, with your foot flexed, and press your heel upward. Hold for about 10 full breaths, or as long as you can. Release, then switch legs and repeat.

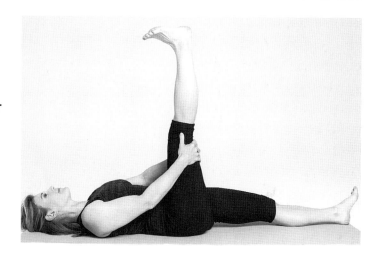

3. Child's Pose

Roll over onto your hands and knees, then lower your hips so they rest on your heels. Reach your arms out in front of you, palms down. Lean forward and gently lower your forehead to the floor, rounding your spine and shoulders. Allow your body to relax completely as you breathe deeply and slowly. Stay in this pose for 10 full breaths, or as long as you can.

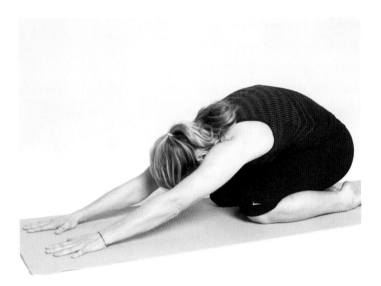

4. Pigeon Stretch

Kneel on all fours, then extend your right leg behind you as far as possible and lower your chest as far as you can toward your left thigh. If possible, turn your left heel in toward your right hip. Press back with the ball of the right foot while pushing through your heel. Hold for about 10 full breaths, or as long as you can. Breathe deeply and switch to the other side.

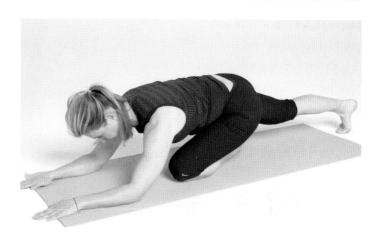

5. Kneeling Arm Stretch with Kegels

Kneel on the floor with your back tall and straight. Gently press your hips back to sit on your heels. Interlace your fingers behind you and press up and back, stretching your shoulders and upper back. Close your eyes and breathe through the stretch. Do 20 Kegels as you hold the stretch.

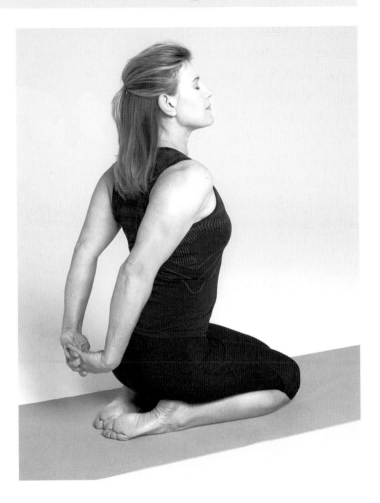

6. Downward Dog

Kneel on all fours with your hands under your shoulders and your knees in line with your hips. Keeping your hands pressed into the floor, straighten your legs and lift your hips up to the ceiling. Your body should look like an inverted V. Press your hands and heels down into the floor and lift your tailbone so you feel a deep stretch in the backs of your legs. Continue pressing down with your hands and heels as you breathe deeply. Hold for 5 to 8 full breaths, or as long as you can. Slowly walk your hands toward your feet as you lift your heels off the floor and bend your knees slightly. Next, slowly walk your hands up your legs and lift your torso to return to an upright standing position.

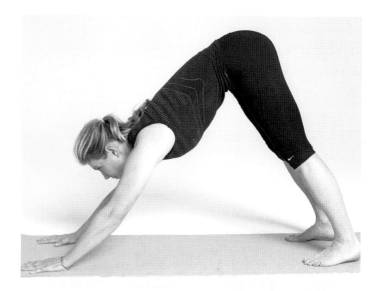

7. Side Lunge Stretch

Take a big step to the right with your right foot, toes pointed to the side. Your left toes should point forward. Bend your right knee into a lunge, so your right knee is directly over your right ankle. Exhale and lower your right hand to the ground. At the same time, extend your left arm up toward the ceiling. Look at your left hand extended way above you. Open your chest and breathe. Feel your shoulders open. Stay in this position for 5 to 8 full breaths, or as long as you can. Slowly return to the starting position. Repeat on the other side.

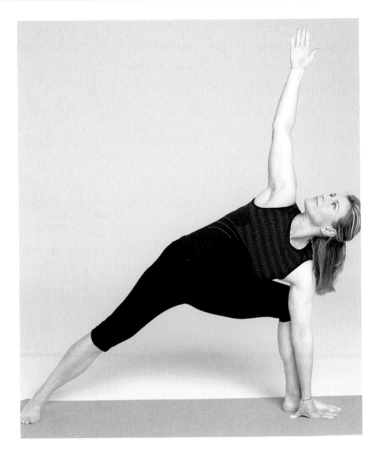

8. Quiet Breath

Stand tall with your feet flat on the floor and your hands resting on your hips. Close your eyes. Listen to the sounds around you. Slowly breathe in through your nose and out through your nose. Do this a few times. Now breathe in through your nose and out your mouth with an *aaaahhhhh* sound. Do this a few times. Now stand quietly for a few moments. Relish this time that is yours.

3

. . . .

Take-Five
Workouts

N o QUESTION, the physical changes that come with getting older can be a drag. But you don't have to let them control your life. In the time it takes you to grab a cup of coffee, throw a load of laundry in the washer, or flip through the channels looking for something to watch on TV, you can do one of my Take-Five Workouts. Each of these five-minute routines is designed to address a different age-related symptom, including sleep deprivation, fatigue, hot flashes, and a sluggish sex drive. While I refer to them as workouts, some involve exercises for your mind instead of your body. Do them whenever and wherever the need arises!

Boost Your Libido

For some women, sex gets better with age. For others, it becomes about as fun and exciting as a fireworks display in the middle of the afternoon. Thanks to waning hormones, lack of energy, or stress—or all of the above—many of us just don't have the spontaneous sexual desire that we used to. If you're feeling sexually uninterested or have a case of the blahs, try doing the following yoga routine with your partner. It can help ignite the passion by providing an opportunity to touch, talk, and relax together. Even if it doesn't lead to a night of wild sex, it can make you feel closer and more connected.

Find a spot in your home where you both have enough room to do the poses. You can use yoga mats or towels on the carpet. Comfortable clothing is critical. Music can also help you get in the mood. I have two favorite CDs: *Simple Things* by Zero 7, a British duo that combines soul music and funk, and Brazilian siren Bebel Gilberto's self-titled collection, which has a slinky samba groove. Use this meditative time to appreciate the special qualities your partner brings to your relationship. Stay close to each other to feel your togetherness. Become more in tune with each other as you move through the poses. Add some kissing and caressing, and who knows—sparks could fly!

1. Moon Pose

Stand side by side, holding hands. Then step about 3 feet away from each other. Standing tall, exhale as you both take your outside arm up and overhead. Side bend toward your partner, allowing your hips to move slightly away from each other. Clasp hands with your partner above your heads. Breathe into your belly and ribs on the outside of your body. Stay in the pose for 5 full breaths. Switch sides and repeat.

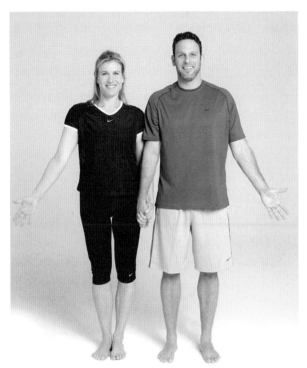 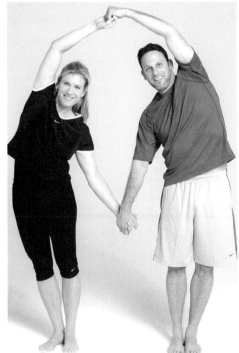

2. Padahastasana

Stand back to back about 1 foot away from each other. Reach back and hold hands. Inhale and stand tall. Exhale as you slowly flex forward from your hips into a forward bend, keeping your legs straight. Stop halfway down, gently pull on each other's arms, lengthen your chest, and press your buttocks into your partner's. Maintain contact. As you sink deeper into the forward bend, gradually move your hands up until you're holding your partner's forearms. Hold for 5 full breaths. Slowly lift your torso to return to the starting position.

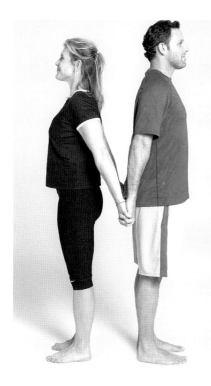

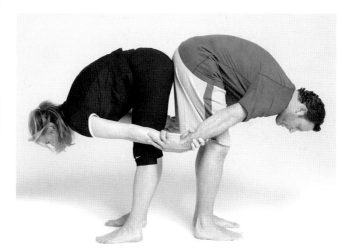

3. Warrior

Start by standing one behind the other in a mountain pose: Stand tall with your feet together, your arms by your sides, your abs pulled in, and your shoulders back. Step your feet 4 to 5 feet apart and turn your right foot out 90 degrees and your left foot in slightly. Lift your arms straight out to the sides at shoulder height, with your palms facing down. Exhale and bend your right leg so that your knee is in line with your ankle and your right thigh is parallel to the floor. Turn your head so you're looking down the length of your right arm, reaching back slightly with your left arm. Hold for 5 full breaths. On the last inhale, come up to the center and repeat on the other side.

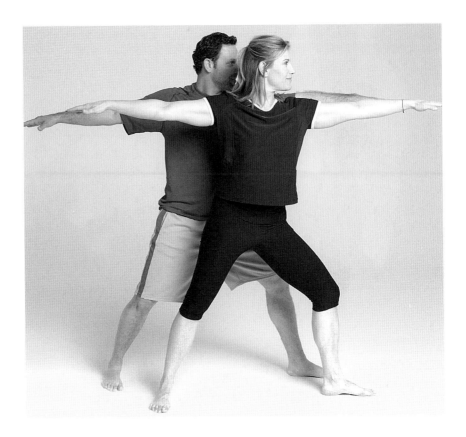

4. Downward Dog

Start by kneeling on all fours; your partner should stand facing you with his feet near your hands. Drop your forehead to the floor. Push up into downward dog, straightening your legs and lifting your tailbone to the ceiling. Your back should be flat and your heels as close to the floor as possible. Your partner should place his toes on top of your hands and lean forward to gently press down on your lower back to intensify the stretch. You should feel the stretch in your hamstrings. Hold the pose for 5 full breaths, then bend your knees to return to the starting position. Switch positions and repeat.

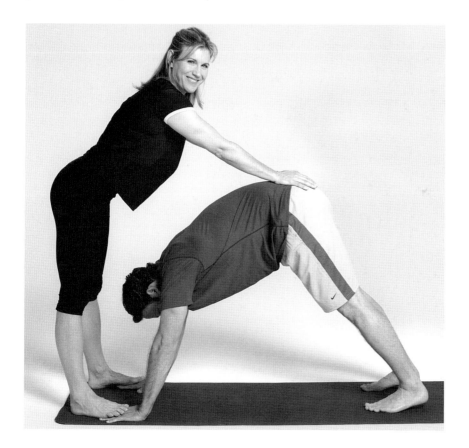

5. Hug

Stand face-to-face and wrap your arms around each other. Place your head on each other's shoulders and breathe. Take deep breaths and long exhalations. Feel each other's warmth. Stay in this position for 5 full breaths, or as long as you want.

Beat the Heat

Hot flashes, hot flushes, power surges, the eternal summer—regardless of what you call them, these sudden waves of intense heat are no fun. And they can strike at the most inopportune times, leaving you with a bright red face or covered in perspiration. What's a girl to do? Start by implementing the strategies on page 18, which included dressing in layers and avoiding spicy foods. In addition, do the following deep breathing and visualization routine twice a day, and whenever you feel a hot flash coming on.

Grab a cold glass of water and retreat to a quiet spot in your home or office. If possible, close the door, turn off the phone, and sit in a comfortable chair or on the floor on a yoga pillow or cushion. Take a sip of the water and begin to slowly breathe in and out. Focus on your breath. Visualize yourself being alone in a cool place, such as a waterfall. Picture the heat escaping through your hands and feet.

Next, imagine taking off your shoes and feel the cool water splashing at your toes and up onto your ankles. Take a deep breath into your belly. There isn't a person in sight. As you stand alone at the water's edge, picture an ice sculpture floating in the water toward you. On the ice sculpture are two trees with a hammock hung in the middle. Notice the chill of the sculpture as it approaches. Slowly and carefully step onto the sculpture and lie in the hammock. Feel the coolness of the ice enveloping your body. Listen to the water lapping the shore as you float away into a chilly dream state.

Feel your heart rate slowing. Feel the calming of your body and your soul. Let go of the tension. Let go of your stress. Let go of the heat. Feel the coolness on the small of your back and the nape of your neck. Be still and breathe. Stay in this cool spot for 5 minutes, or until your hot flash passes.

Head Off an Emotional Blowout

How many times have you almost lost it . . . with either your kids, your husband, your co-workers, or the innocent telemarketer who calls when you're in the middle of dinner? It happens to me more often than I'd like to admit. For whatever reason, I lose my patience. I snap, I get mean, I yell. The littlest thing can set me over the edge, and all the uglies come whirling out. After the fact, my husband, Billy, often asks me, "Do you know what a bitch you can be? Why do you do this?" But I can't explain why it happens. It just does. It must be those wacky hormones.

Recently, though, I've found a supereffective—albeit unconventional—way to defuse my time bomb before it explodes. Whenever I feel my blood starting to boil, I stand on my head. Yes, you heard me right. Crazy as it sounds, doing a simple headstand helps calm me down instantly. Because it requires balance and focus, it takes my mind off my frustrations and forces me to let go of my anger.

Headstands have been around since ancient times. In yoga, the headstand is known as the "King of Asanas" because of its many benefits. When you stand on your head, you reverse the effects of gravity. This lessens the strain on your heart and allows a fresh supply of blood to flow to your brain. It is a centering, calming, and soothing pose that can help relieve stress and mild depression. Headstands don't require a great deal of strength. For some of you, the only hard part may be conquering your fear.

When I was a youngster, during gymnastics class I started the headstand from the tripod position. Alternatively, you can do the traditional yoga method. Start by holding the headstand for about 15 to 30 seconds, and gradually work up to 5 minutes or longer. If you're nervous or balance-challenged, do the headstand close to a wall. Headstand supports for your shoulders are available online at www.gaiam.com. Don't do this move if you have high blood pressure or a detached retina, or have experienced neck, back, or shoulder problems.

A word of caution: In yoga, headstands are considered an advanced pose, so if you have not been physically active for a while, start off by doing a tripod headstand against the wall.

From the Tripod Position

Squat on an exercise mat and place your hands in front of you on the mat about shoulder width apart. Curl over to rest the top of your head on the mat in front of your hands to form an equilateral triangle. Place one knee at a time on top of your elbows. Your center of gravity should be located over the center of the triangle. After you find your balance, slowly extend your legs straight up in the air into a headstand. Hold this position for as long as you can. To come out of the headstand, you can either bend your knees back to tripod position or shift your weight forward, place your chin on your chest, round your back, and roll forward and back up onto your feet.

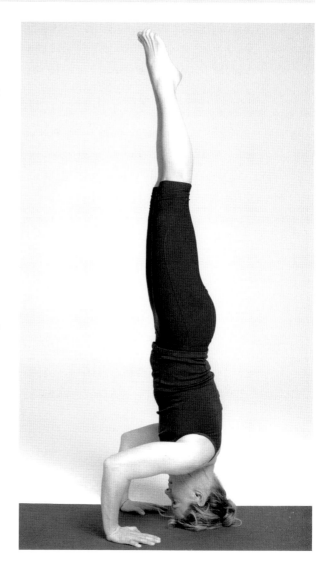

Traditional Yoga Headstand

Kneel on the exercise mat with your buttocks resting on your heels. Lean forward and place your forearms in front of you on the mat, about shoulder width apart. Interlace your fingers, tucking your pinky fingers underneath. Place the top of your head on the mat and press the back of your head against the inside of your interlocked fingers. Now, straighten your legs and lift your hips as if you were coming into downward dog. Without bending your knees, walk your feet in as close as possible to your head. Pull your hips back so that your neck is aligned with your spine. Bend your knees into your chest and lift your feet off the floor. Keeping your knees bent, use your abs to lift your legs straight up toward the ceiling. Reach up through the balls of your feet and rotate your thigh bones inward slightly. Hold for as long as you can, then reverse the steps to lower yourself back down to the mat.

Sleep Like a Baby

Remember the days when you could sleep for eight blissful, uninterrupted hours? Our bodies still need those ZZZZs, but getting them isn't so easy. Between anxiety and night sweats and those middle-of-the-night trips to the bathroom, many of us wind up counting *a lot* of sheep. Well, it's time to take back our nights. The following bedtime routine will help you unwind, soothe your mind, and gently prepare your body for sleep. It works for me, and it will work for you. You'll awake refreshed and ready to start a new day. Sweet dreams!

1. Legs on the Wall

This stretch can help relieve the tension from a long day of standing or running around. Your legs will love it, especially if you have leg cramps or varicose veins.

Lie on your back with your legs extended straight up against a wall and your buttocks as close to the base of the wall as possible. (To get into this position, try sitting with your right side close to a wall, then lying back and pivoting your hips to the right as you extend your legs straight up.) Your arms should be by your sides, with your palms facing up. Keep your legs straight and turn your focus to your breathing. Close your eyes and feel the air fill your body as you breathe in and out. Relax and enjoy the moment. Stay in this position for 1 minute or even longer, if you can.

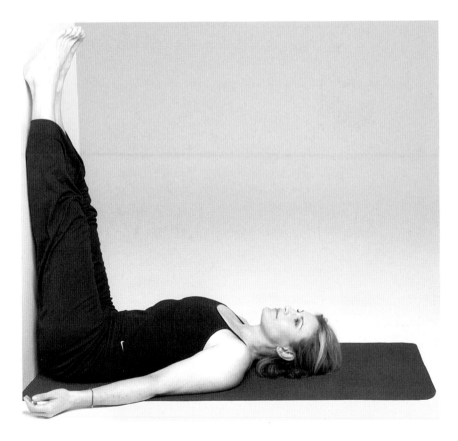

2. Pretzel Stretch

Lie on your back about a foot and a half from the wall. Bring both knees into your chest. Cross your right thigh over your left and position your legs so that both knees form right angles. Hold your ankles and pull your legs toward your chest. Hold for about 30 seconds, then switch legs and repeat.

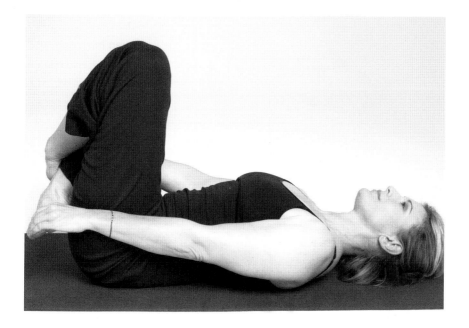

3. Side-to-Side Stretch

This stretch will soothe your back.

Pull your knees in toward your chest. Gently drop your knees to the right. Extend your left arm so it is stretched out to the side. Gently press down on your legs with your right hand for a deeper stretch. Hold the twist for 5 slow, deep breaths. Switch sides and repeat.

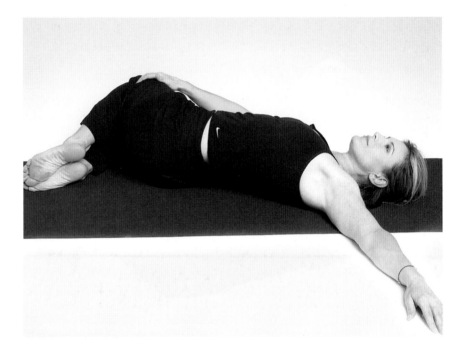

4. Ujjayi Breath

If you've taken a yoga class, you may be familiar with Ujjayi breathing. Also called ocean-sounding breath, it can help still your mind, relax your body, and increase blood flow to your lungs and heart.

Lie on your back with your knees bent and your feet flat on the floor. Put your right hand on your heart and your left hand on your lower belly. Inhale deeply with your mouth closed and your throat as open as possible. You will make the sound of the ocean similar to what you hear in a conch shell. Pick a spot on the ceiling to focus on. Your breath should be seamless. Feel your belly expand and empty with each breath. Stay in this pose for at least 1 minute.

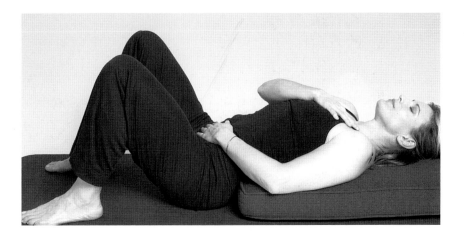

5. Butterfly Stretch

This stretch eases stress and opens your hips and chest. Use a blanket for extra cushioning. This is *soooo* comfortable; make sure you don't end up sleeping on the floor for the night!

Lie on your back with a folded blanket or towel under the base of your spine, hands resting by your sides, palms facing up. Bring the bottoms of your feet together and let your knees flop out to the sides. Imagine you're floating through the air and feel your breath moving throughout your body. Let the tension go. With each breath, feel your muscles sink deeper and deeper into the floor. Stay here for 1 minute, or as long as you can. You'll love the way this feels. Just make sure you make it back to your bed for a dreamy night of slumber.

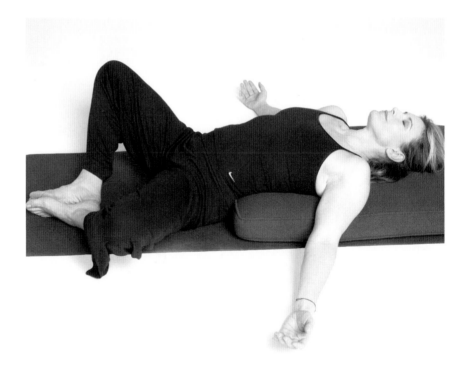

Regain Your Energy

The stress, the sleepless nights, the emotional tirades. No wonder you feel tired all the time! Believe me, I can relate. Sometimes I just feel like curling up on the couch and closing my eyes, or grabbing a diet soda to keep me going. But instead, a little movement is exactly what I need. Research shows that even 5 minutes of physical activity can effectively boost your energy. So whenever you're feeling sluggish, try this quick pick-me-up. It will help transport blood and oxygen to your muscles and your brain to revive your body. Do each of the following exercises for 1 minute, and you should feel ready to tackle the rest of your day.

1. Straight Leg Kicks

Stand tall with your feet hip width apart,
your hands on your hips. Kick your right
leg in front of you to about hip height; at
the same time, reach out with your left
hand and touch your toes. Keep your abs
pulled in tightly and your upper body upright. Repeat with the opposite leg and
arm. Continue alternating sides for
1 minute. *If you can't touch your toes
on the first few kicks, reach as far as you
can. As your body warms up, you should
feel more flexible, so continue trying to
touch them.*

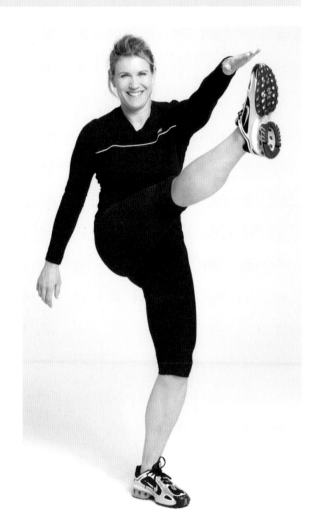

2. Touch Down Reverse Lunges

Stand tall with your feet hip width apart. Step backward with your right foot and bend both knees into a lunge. Your left knee should be directly over your left ankle, your right heel lifted. Touch the floor with your right hand close to the inside of your left foot. Straighten your legs to return to the starting position. Repeat, stepping back with your left foot. Continue alternating legs for 1 minute.

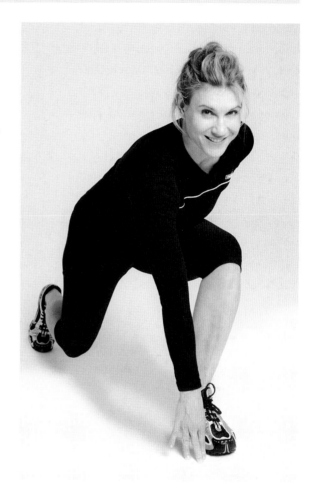

3. Butt Squat

Stand with your feet hip width apart. Keeping your abs pulled in tight, bend your knees to lower yourself down into a squat, keeping your knees slightly in front of your ankles and your weight on your heels. Do 2 sets of 10.

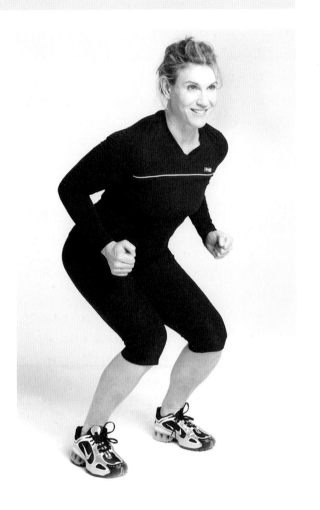

4. Tricep Dips

Sit on a sturdy chair with your hands on the front edge of the seat, fingers facing forward. Supporting yourself on your hands, walk your feet forward so your butt is just in front of the chair seat, knees straight. Your back should be close to the chair. Bend your elbows to lower yourself down toward the floor, until your elbows are just above your shoulders. Exhale as you use your arms to press back up to the starting position. Do this for 1 minute.

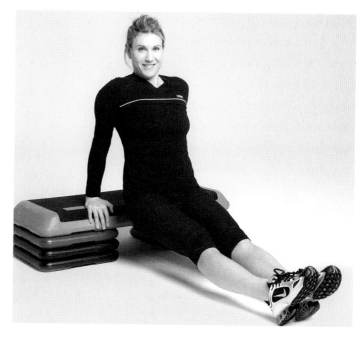

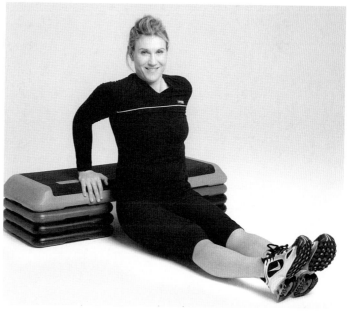

5. Ab Pull-Ups

Sit on the edge of the chair with your hands wrapped around the sides of the chair seat. Lean back and extend your toes to the floor with a slight bend in your knees. Lean your upper body back into the chair. Exhale and tighten your abs as you curl your upper body forward and pull your knees in toward your chest. Return to the starting position. Do this for 1 minute.

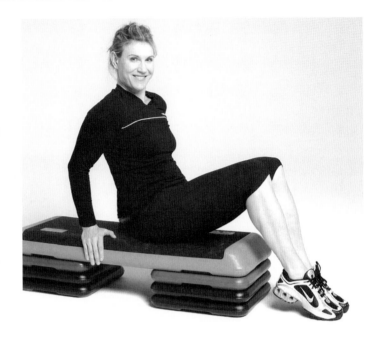

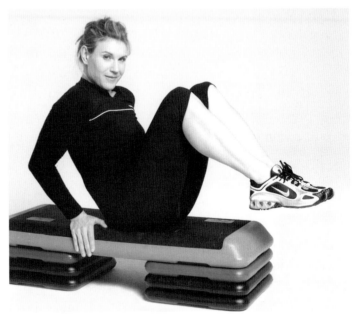

4

. . . .

A New Plan
for Nourishing
Your Body

EVERY CHAPTER of your life comes with its own unique nutritional requirements. That's because as we grow older, our bodies have different needs. And while I know you've been enjoying a healthy diet up until this point (I'm giving you the benefit of the doubt here!), you may need to update your eating habits to include certain foods and exclude others to keep yourself in top shape.

Like it or not, our bodies are changing. Our metabolisms are slowing down. You may have already noticed a few more curves where you'd rather not notice them. Maybe you're feeling a little bloated. And perhaps you've experienced a hot flash or two. My nutritional plan will help you tackle these midlife challenges and more.

As you know, your eating habits can help or hurt you when it comes to bolstering your body against heart disease, cancer, osteoporosis, and diabetes. In this chapter, I'll explain which foods and nutrients can protect you from these ravages of aging. But don't worry: I'm not about to overwhelm you with dozens of dietary "dos" and "don'ts." Instead, I've streamlined my plan into just five simple goals. By making these five changes to your diet, you can dramatically improve your health.

Just to clarify: This isn't a diet book. On the following pages, you won't find structured meal plans or detailed grocery lists. I'm not going to tell you to count calories or avoid pasta like the plague. And I won't promise that you'll drop ten pounds in a week. But here's what I can guarantee: By following my easy eating strategies, you *can* control your weight, energize your body, and add years to your life. Best of all, you won't have to go hungry or give up your favorite foods.

I must confess: Healthy eating hasn't always come easily to me. In fact, from my late teens and through my twenties, I struggled terribly with food. My battle began in high school, when I began taking over-the-counter diet pills to lose weight. I brought this terrible habit with me to college, where I also became bulimic. On a typical day, I would take a diet pill, go without food until I was absolutely famished, then binge and purge.

To put it mildly, my body paid the price. My sophomore year in college, I suffered a grand mal seizure, which landed me in the hospital and scared me to death. Still, for whatever reason, it wasn't enough to make me stop. I continued in the vicious binge–purge–diet pill cycle for another year, until I had a second seizure. This one finally knocked some sense into me. I vowed to stop taking diet pills and throwing up, and to start eating right.

I maintained my good habits for about six years, until I moved to Los Angeles. On the surface, my life was going great; my personal training career was flourishing and I was dating a famous actor. But I wasn't taking care of myself. I was overexercising, undereating, drinking tons of coffee, and not sleeping enough. Before long, my foolish ways caught up with me again. In 1990, I suffered another seizure while hiking with a client. My physician threatened to put me on antiseizure medication, which meant that my driver's license would be revoked. I knew I had to make a major change. My livelihood—not to mention my life—depended on it. So once again I cleaned up my act—and this time, it was for good. I finally learned how to eat in a way that nourished and nurtured my body.

These days, I don't follow any strict rules or use a scale to measure portions. I practice moderation and eat a variety of foods—including pesto pasta, cheese pizza, and Nutella, every once in a while. Eating is one of life's greatest pleasures. I truly believe that you should allow yourself to indulge in the foods that you love, and do it without guilt. Eating small amounts of these foods isn't going to kill you. What it *will* do is satisfy your cravings, so you're less likely to go overboard.

In other words, I've developed an eating style that's more relaxed, balanced, and, well, mature. Because let's face it: If a diet plan is too complicated and restrictive, you're not going to stick with it. You need the simplicity, reality, and sensibility of my plan, not the extremes of some of today's crazy diet schemes.

While I'm not a nutritionist, I know what works for me. To put together this chapter, I also consulted with some of the top experts in the field, including my friend Carolyn O'Neil, RD, co-author of *The Dish on Eating Healthy and Being Fabulous!* (Atria Books, June 2004). So follow my guidelines and let common sense prevail!

Goal #1: Go Au Naturel

I know what you're thinking, but I'm not about to tell you to parade around in the buff. (Though that certainly would inspire most people to watch what they eat!) I'm talking about filling up with wholesome, natural foods as much as you can. By wholesome and natural, I mean foods that are nutritious and aren't loaded with added sugars, salt, and strange chemicals that you can't even pronounce.

If you follow this simple rule, you should automatically find yourself reaching for more fruits and vegetables, which are low in calories and filled with antioxidants. Research shows that a diet packed with fresh

An Apple a Day Keeps the Menopot Away!

That's right, the same fruit that supposedly keeps the doctor away also may help keep your bulging belly at bay. It's been my favorite weight control secret for years. Apples are rich in pectin, a soluble fiber that's a natural appetite suppressant. How does it work? The pectin slows down your digestive process, which makes you feel fuller, longer. At only 80 calories for a medium-sized apple, it is the best multitasking snack out there. It tastes great, fills you up, and nourishes your body with vitamins and fiber. Try munching an apple midmorning so you're not starving at lunch, or in the late afternoon to keep you from going overboard at dinner.

fruits and veggies can decrease your risk of cardiovascular disease. One study of 110,000 men and women found that those who averaged eight or more servings a day cut their risk of heart attack and stroke by 30 percent. Boosting your intake of fruits and vegetables may also help ward off certain cancers, including lung, ovary, colon, stomach, and mouth cancer, and guard against cataracts and macular degeneration, two common causes of vision loss.

Along with fruits and veggies, you should strive to eat more whole grains, including oatmeal and whole wheat bread, which are a great source of micronutrients such as folic acid, magnesium, and vitamin E, all of which have been shown to help prevent heart disease and diabetes. Certain cancer risks are also reduced when you dine on whole grains.

And let's not forget nuts and legumes, another natural source of protein, vitamins, and minerals. Nuts, which contain mostly unsaturated fats (the healthy kind!) along with vitamin E, folic acid, potassium, and other nutrients, have been linked to a lower risk of heart disease. In fact, some varieties (including walnuts, almonds, pecans, peanuts, hazelnuts, and pistachios) are now allowed to carry a claim that eating an ounce a day can protect your heart. Legumes—a class of vegetables that includes soybeans, black beans, lima beans, peas, and lentils—are typically low in fat and rich in folate, potassium, iron, and magnesium. Like other vegetables, they contain phytochemicals, plant compounds that may help prevent cardiovascular disease, cancer, and other diseases.

All of these nourishing foods—fruits, veggies, whole grains, nuts, and legumes—also supply dietary fiber to help keep your weight in check. Because it absorbs water as it passes through your digestive tract, fiber helps fill you up, so you're more likely to feel satisfied before you've eaten too much. Fiber also whisks other food through your system, so your body absorbs fewer calories. A high-fiber diet can reduce your risk of developing diabetes and also lower your blood cholesterol level to protect your heart. And as we all know, fiber can help fight constipation, one of my least favorite side effects of getting older.

Of course, I know it isn't always easy to eat this way, especially when you're on the run. The last time I hit a fast-food restaurant, there wasn't a single fresh fruit, vegetable, or whole grain on the menu! Not to worry, though, one less-nutritious lunch won't undo a week's worth of healthy eating. But if you plan ahead, you can make it easier to achieve this goal. For starters, make sure your kitchen is stocked with wholesome snacks. Keep unsalted nuts in your desk drawer so you avoid the vending machine when you're starving. Pack a lunch if you plan to be out running around all day. Adjust your driving route to pass by a natural foods store. It may take a little extra effort, but the payoff will be worth it.

Goal #2: Take a Lump out of Your Sugar Habit

If you're worried about your waistline—and let's face it, who isn't?—one of the smartest things that you can do is cut back on sweets. Whenever I'm trying to slim down for a TV appearance or a photo shoot, I make an extra effort to forgo them. Why? Unlike the natural sugars found in fresh fruits, vegetables, and milk products, which are packed with vitamins and minerals, the refined sugars in cookies, candy, ice cream, fruit juices, and sodas are essentially "empty" calories that do little to nourish your body. Plus they can trigger a sudden increase in blood sugar that causes you to overeat.

Here's how it works: When you wolf down a sugary treat, such as a donut or candy bar, your blood sugar rises quickly, prompting your body to secrete large amounts of insulin in an effort to stabilize it. This surge in insulin causes your blood sugar to plummet again, which can leave you feeling irritable and sluggish. So you reach for another snack to get you going again. It's a vicious circle.

In recent years, research has demonstrated that having a sweet tooth can translate to extra inches. In one study published in the prestigious *Journal of the American Medical Association,* middle-aged women who drank one or more sugar-sweetened beverages (soda or fruit juice, for example) per day gained an average of more than seventeen pounds over an eight-year period. Their counterparts who were instructed to drink no more than one sugary drink each week also gained some weight—but only about six pounds on average.

The U.S. Department of Agriculture (USDA) recommends that the average person on a 2,000-calorie-per-day diet limit added sugars to 40 grams a day. That's approximately ten teaspoons. Ten teaspoons sounds like a lot until you realize it's the amount in one twelve-ounce can of Pepsi, a quarter cup of pancake syrup, or a small piece of pumpkin pie. Yikes! What can you do? Start by curbing your intake of candy, cookies, cakes, pies, soft drinks, ice cream, and other obvious offenders. Then keep an eye out for hidden sources, including breakfast cereals, pasta sauces, flavored yogurts, peanut butter, dried fruits, and bread products.

I call these *stealth sugars*—and the only way to avoid them is to know where they are. So start reading the labels on all the foods you buy. Look for terms that indicate added sugars, such as sucrose, fructose, high-fructose corn syrup, glucose, dextrose, and maltose. Don't be fooled by healthy-sounding ingredients such as honey, brown rice syrup, and evaporated cane juice. They may be more natural, but they're no more nourishing than white sugar—and they still contain unnecessary calories. A basic rule of thumb: If sugar or some other sweetener is one of the top three ingredients, or the product lists more than one source of sugar, think twice.

Now I'm certainly not saying that you can never enjoy a chocolate bar or a slice of cheesecake ever again. What kind of life would that be? You just don't want to do it all the time. So examine your diet and see where you can lose some extra sugar. If you crave a sweet at the end of your meal, try some unsweetened applesauce or a decaf soy latte sprinkled with cinnamon. Swap the flavored yogurt for plain yogurt topped with fresh berries. Skip the chocolate chip cookie and eat a graham cracker instead. Dying for a soda? Sip some flavored seltzer with a twist of lime. Rather than cake, bake a loaf of pumpkin bread and reduce the sugar in the recipe by a third. If you're a sugar addict, you might miss the sweetness at first. But after a week, I bet you won't crave it at all—and you'll absolutely love the way you feel.

The 90/10 Rule

Believe me, I love sweets and junk food, just like everyone else. And I know that totally depriving myself of these treats is a recipe for overindulging. So I've adopted what I call the 90/10 rule. Ninety percent of the time, I consume lots of fresh fruits, vegetables, whole grains, and lean protein, and limit fatty and sugary foods. The other 10 percent of the time, I eat whatever I want, whether it's some Flamin' Hot Cheetos (my kids are addicted to them!), a side of curly fries, or a Diet Coke. As long as you stick to my simple 90/10 guideline—and watch your portion sizes—you'll be in good shape!

Goal #3: Mooo-re Calcium

Remember when Mom told you to drink your milk for strong bones? Well, that advice holds true today. The calcium found in dairy products as well as in leafy green vegetables and other foods is essential for slowing the bone loss that can start as early as our thirties and accelerates in the years immediately following menopause. Unless you take steps to combat it, this deterioration can lead to broken bones and spinal fractures that cause loss of mobility, shrinking stature, and a hunched back— a condition otherwise known as osteoporosis.

While we tend to think of bones as inert, they are actually living tissues that are constantly changing. Every minute of every day, calcium is deposited into and removed from our bones to build them up and break them down. Sometime after age thirty, due to inadequate intake of calcium, inactivity, and hormonal changes, our bones begin breaking down faster than they build up. When we hit menopause and our estrogen production plummets, we start losing bone even faster. It's been estimated that the average woman loses 3 to 5 percent of her bone mass each year in the first five years after menopause. Eventually, it starts to ease up again. But by then, many of us are on the slippery slope to osteoporosis.

Boosting your calcium intake is one simple step you can take to combat this bone blitz. If you're under age fifty, experts from the National Institutes of Health (NIH) recommend consuming at least 1,000 milligrams of calcium a day. If you're over age fifty, your goal should be 1,000 milligrams daily if you're taking hormones, and 1,500 milligrams if you're not. Unfortunately, even though we know how important it is, most of us aren't coming close to meeting these requirements. According to the NIH's Office of Dietary Supplements, 78 percent of adult women aren't getting enough of this essential bone-building nutrient.

Eating more calcium-rich foods, particularly low-fat dairy products, is a great place to start. Milk, yogurt, and cheese are some of the rich-

Don't Forget the D!

Calcium is best absorbed when you have an adequate amount of vitamin D in your body. Vitamin D is known as the "sunshine vitamin" because your skin manufactures it after direct exposure to ultraviolet light. Exposing your hands, arms, and face to direct sun—minus the sunscreen—for fifteen minutes, two to three times a week, is usually enough to meet your vitamin D requirement. (Sunscreen, window glass, and clothing diminish the amount of vitamin D manufactured by your skin.) If you're reluctant to go into the sun, make sure your multivitamin or calcium supplement contains vitamin D, and eat plenty of vitamin-D fortified foods such as milk, soy milk, and some breakfast cereals. Vitamin D is also found in small amounts in oily fishes such as salmon and sardines, egg yolks, and liver. Recommended daily intakes are 200 IU for women under age fifty, and 400 IU for women over age fifty.

est sources. Other good ones include salmon, sardines, oysters, spinach, collard greens, and broccoli. Calcium-fortified foods, such as orange juice, soy milk, breakfast cereals, energy bars, and Propel Calcium Fitness Water, can also help you meet your calcium needs.

Theoretically, if you eat a healthy, well-balanced diet, you should be able to meet your daily calcium quota. However, because most of us don't consume enough calcium-rich foods, it's a good idea to take a calcium supplement (along with your multivitamin) to reach the recommended level of 1,000 to 1,500 milligrams per day.

Calcium supplements come in many shapes and sizes. Many women choose Tums, which are available in either 200- or 300-milligram tablets. Caltrate, Os-Cal, and Citracal are other popular brands. There's also my personal favorite, Viactiv Soft Calcium Chews. Each chew contains 20 calories and 500 milligrams of calcium along with vitamins D and K.

How Much Calcium Is There In . . . ?

Food	Amount	Calcium (in milligrams)	Percent Daily Value (DV)
Yogurt, plain, low fat	8 ounces	415	42%
Yogurt, fruit, low fat	8 ounces	245–384	25–38%
Cheddar cheese	1.5 ounces	306	31%
Milk, nonfat	8 fluid ounces	302	30%
Milk, reduced fat (2% milk fat)	8 fluid ounces	297	30%
Mozzarella, part skim	1.5 ounces	275	28%
Tofu, firm, made with calcium sulfate,	½ cup	204	20%
Orange juice, calcium fortified	6 fluid ounces	200–260	20–26%
Cottage cheese, 1% milk fat	1 cup unpacked	138	14%
Tofu, soft, made with calcium sulfate	½ cup	138	14%
Spinach, cooked	½ cup	120	12%
Frozen yogurt, vanilla, soft serve	½ cup	103	10%
Ready-to-eat cereal, calcium fortified	1 cup	100–1,000	10–100%
Turnip greens, boiled	½ cup	99	10%
Kale, cooked	1 cup	94	9%
Soy beverage, calcium fortified	8 fluid ounces	80–500	8–50%

Source: National Institutes of Health Office of Dietary Supplements

They come in four flavors: milk chocolate, caramel, mochaccino, and orange cream.

Because our bodies can absorb only so much calcium at once, experts advise taking no more than 500 milligrams at a time. So if you're aiming for a total of 1,000 milligrams, you'll want to pop your supplements at different times of day—and not in conjunction with your multivitamin. Most calcium supplements contain either calcium carbonate or calcium citrate. If you're taking calcium carbonate (the most common type of calcium supplement), it's best to take it with food, because the acid secreted by your stomach during digestion helps boost absorption. Calcium citrate doesn't need stomach acid to be absorbed, so you can take it at any time. Whatever kind of supplement you choose, follow the instructions on the label.

Bear in mind that while dietary calcium can go a long way in protecting your bones, it may not be enough. At least two studies have shown that increasing calcium intake won't completely offset the bone loss that occurs during menopause. So to keep those bones strong and healthy, be sure to do regular weight-bearing exercise, such as walking and strength training, as well. It's also important to consume less sodium, stop smoking, and avoid excessive alcohol intake—all of which can up your osteoporosis risk.

If you undergo a bone density test and are found to have thinning bones, your doctor may recommend drugs such as bisphosphates or selective estrogen receptor modulators (SERMs), which can help increase calcium intake into your bones. Hormone therapy has also been shown to help prevent bone fractures—though most experts recommend investigating other treatment options before going the hormone route.

Goal #4: Choose Healthy Fats

It's been beaten into our heads for years—fat is *bad, bad, bad*. After all, it can stick to our arteries, add inches to our waist, and take years off our life, right? Well, not exactly. The fact is, there are good fats and bad fats. And while eating too much of the bad kind could increase your risk for heart disease and other health problems, the good fats can—and should—be part of a healthy diet.

Despite its bad rap, fat is vital for energy, satiety, and overall good health. It helps insulate the tissues in our bodies and transport fat-soluble vitamins through our blood. Because it's digested more slowly than either protein or carbohydrates, it helps you feel more content. Fat

Fat: The Good, the Bad, and the Ugly

Type of Fat	Main Source	State at Room Temperature	Effect on Cholesterol Levels
Monounsaturated	Olives; olive oil; canola oil; peanut oil; cashews, almonds, peanuts, and most other nuts; avocados	Liquid	Lowers LDL; raises HDL
Polyunsaturated	Corn, soybean, safflower, and cottonseed oils; fish	Liquid	Lowers LDL; raises HDL
Saturated	Whole milk, butter, cheese, and ice cream; red meat; chocolate; coconuts, coconut milk, and coconut oil	Solid	Raises both LDL and HDL
Trans	Most margarines; vegetable shortening; partially hydrogenated vegetable oil; deep-fried chips; many fast foods; most commercial baked goods	Solid or semisolid	Raises LDL

Source: Harvard School of Public Health Nutrition Source

also helps bring out the flavor in food, which makes it more enjoyable and satisfying.

Unsaturated fats, which typically come from plant sources such as vegetable oils, nuts, and avocados, are the healthy ones that have been shown to lower low-density lipoprotein (LDL) or "bad" cholesterol while increasing high-density lipoprotein (HDL) or "good" cholesterol. The not-so-good kinds include saturated fats—mainly animal fats found in meat, poultry skin, egg yolks, and whole-milk dairy products such as milk, cream, cheese, and butter—which have been shown to raise both LDL and HDL cholesterol. Even worse are trans fats, found in most margarines, vegetable shortening, fried foods, and processed snack foods made with hydrogenated vegetable oils, which raise LDL cholesterol but don't boost HDL.

The bottom line: To keep your heart healthy, strive to consume more unsaturated fats, while limiting saturated fats and avoiding trans fats. Does this mean you can never have a cheeseburger and fries again? Not at all, but you certainly can't afford to eat like that every day. No one can. So instead of a cheeseburger, consider a turkey or chicken burger. They're much lower in saturated fat, are just as tasty, and can be found just about anywhere traditional hamburgers are offered. Craving fries? Make a healthy version by slicing up potatoes, coating them lightly with olive oil, and roasting them in the oven.

And remember, this isn't an excuse to smother your salad with olive oil or eat guacamole by the truckload. All fats—including the unsaturated kind—are a significant source of calories, and will cause you to gain weight if you eat them in excess. So don't overdo it!

Goal #5: Eat Like Clockwork

If, like many women, you associated weight loss with deprivation, you'll be happy to learn that one of my best stay-slim secrets involves eating more often. That's right: Over the years, research has shown that consuming a small meal or snack every few hours can help prevent dips in blood sugar that cause you to overeat. It can also help keep your metabolism charged, so you burn more calories throughout the day.

Want proof? In one recent study published in the journal *Medicine and Science in Sport and Exercise*, researchers from Georgia State University's Laboratory for Elite Athlete Performance in Atlanta examined the eating habits of sixty-eight female athletes over a three-year period. In the end, the women who ate evenly and consistently throughout the day had significantly lower levels of body fat than those who skipped

The Healing Power of Food

Although we all love to celebrate birthdays, as the number of candles on our cake increases, so do the "discomforts" of aging. What and how you eat can make a difference in eliminating or reducing the following side effects.

The Problem	Say "Yes" To . . .	Say "No" To . . .
Headaches	Magnesium-rich foods, such as almonds, barley, and black beans, which have been shown to prevent hormone-induced headaches	Cured meats such as ham and bologna, aged cheeses, monosodium glutamate (MSG), and alcohol (especially red wine)
Bloating	Grapefruit juice, a natural diuretic that helps flush excess water from your system (Caution: Because grapefruit juice can interfere with the absorption of certain drugs, check with your doctor first if you're taking medication.)	High-sodium foods, such as many frozen dinners, canned soups, and packaged snacks
Forgetfulness	Blueberries and other purple fruits and veggies, which contain powerful antioxidants that may help slow or reverse age-related memory loss	Skipping meals; without a steady supply of carbohydrates—your brain's main fuel supply—your memory and concentration will suffer

meals. The longer that certain athletes went without food, the higher their body fat percentages were.

Eating at regular intervals from sunup to sundown will not only help in your fight against middle-age spread: By keeping your blood sugar stable, it can help prevent those wicked mood swings that are all too common during this hormonally charged time of life. You'll also have a steady flow of energy for your workouts and whatever else comes your way.

The Problem	Say "Yes" To . . .	Say "No" To . . .
Hot flashes	Soy foods, such as tofu, edamame, and veggie burgers; they contain substances called phytoestrogens that may help keep hot flashes at bay	Spicy foods, hot drinks, red wine and other alcoholic beverages
Mood swings	Asparagus, beets, Brussels sprouts, bok choy, and other foods rich in B vitamins (including B_6, B_{12}, and folic acid), which have been shown to help relieve depression	Sugary foods, such as cookies, donuts, and candy, which can cause a quick rise and fall in blood sugar that leave you feeling grouchy
Achy joints	Salmon and other oily fishes—preliminary research shows that their omega-3 fatty acids may help reduce joint tenderness and stiffness	Coffee and other caffeinated drinks; they rob your body of water, which can aggravate sore joints and muscles
Bad eyesight	Dark, leafy greens—they contain lutein, an antioxidant that has been shown to ward off age-related macular degeneration (ARMD), the most common cause of vision loss in women over age sixty	Fatty red meat; in one study of 2,000 people age forty-five and older, those who ate the most saturated fat and cholesterol had an 80 percent greater risk of developing ARMD

To make it work, you'll need to watch the clock. Your goal should be to eat something every three to four hours. Don't wait for those hunger pangs to hit! The idea is to never let yourself get too hungry or too full. To get in the habit, you may want to schedule your snack breaks just as you would a doctor's appointment. For example, tell yourself that 10:00 a.m. is snack time and, no matter where you are, have a quick nibble.

Kathy's Favorite Ways to Stay Hydrated

1. Drink and drive. Keep a case of bottled water in the trunk or backseat of your car. That's what actress Penelope Ann Miller, my longtime client, taught me to do. This way, you won't be tempted a grab a cola or other beverage that may sound thirst-quenching, but really makes you more dehydrated or is loaded with empty calories. If you prefer cold water, put your stash in a cooler, or stop at a drive-thru for a cup of ice.

2 Fill an ice cube tray with cranberry, lemon, and lime juice and freeze. This way, you can drop in a cube to add flavor and color to your water.

3. Drink a glass of water before each meal. Aside from keeping you hydrated, it will help quell those hunger pangs so you don't overeat. Ask your server for water as soon as you are seated at a restaurant and try to finish the glass before you order.

4. Cool down with frozen fruit pops made from 100% juice with no added sugar or try Propel Fitness Water for fewer calories. They are mainly water and can help with hot flashes.

5. Increase your intake of water-filled foods, such as watermelon, grapes, tomatoes, zucchini, and low-sodium soups.

To keep your calories in check, watch your portion sizes. Each mini-meal or snack should be small and nutritious. Approach each one as if you're eating only to tide yourself over for a few hours. Instead of devouring a huge sandwich, eat half and save the rest for a snack. If you're dining at a restaurant, ask for a doggie bag and turn the leftovers into tomorrow's lunch.

To get a proper balance of nutrients and keep myself satisfied, I make a conscious effort to include a protein with a complex carbohydrate every time. Here are some of my favorite combinations:

- Half of an apple or a banana with a tablespoon of natural peanut butter

- Cottage cheese with whole-grain crackers

- Freshly cut veggies dipped in hummus

- A hard-boiled egg with Wasa bread crackers

- Sliced turkey with whole wheat pita chips

- A smoothie made with fresh fruit and nonfat milk

- Cucumbers and hummus on whole wheat bread

- Grilled chicken over mixed greens

- High-fiber cereal with plain yogurt

Because I'm constantly on the move—driving to meet a client, flying to New York for the *Today* show, or shuttling my kids around town—I try to keep a stash of healthy snacks with me at all times. Sometimes I put them in a cooler in my car. Other times, I just stick them in my purse or gym bag. Sure, it's easier to say I'll just grab something when I'm out. But as you know, the choices out there in the real world aren't always good for your body.

Drink to Your Health!

1. Want to lose weight? The best drink: vegetable juice.

According to Barbara Rolls, PhD, a Pennsylvania State University professor and co-author of *The Volumetrics Weight-Control Plan: Feel Full on Fewer Calories,* drinking a glass of vegetable juice fifteen to twenty minutes before a meal can reduce the number of calories you eat. The reason is still largely a puzzle, but she suspects that the drink's thickness and calorie density may play a role. Because vegetable juice can be packed with sodium, choose a low-sodium version. One of my favorites is Kagome's True Vegetable Garden (www.kagome.us), which is low in sodium and has no added sugar.

2. Want a kick-butt workout? The best drink: green tea.

A study published in the *Journal of the American Physiological Society* found that green tea extract improved exercise endurance up to 24 percent and increased the amount of fat burned. The research, which was conducted on mice swimming in a pool, found that those given the extract tired less easily over the ten-week period and had higher rates of fat oxidation. While more research is needed to prove the theory, the study's lead author believes that drinking a few cups of green tea before a workout should have similar effects in humans.

3. Want to raise your glass without going overboard on calories? The best drink: vodka tonic.

If you want to enjoy an occasional cocktail without packing on the pounds, remember that the blander and clearer the drink, the fewer the calories. Stick with clear spirits, such as vodka and gin—both of which have about 100 calories in a 1.5-ounce serving—mixed with a no-cal mixer such as club soda or diet tonic water. By comparison, a 6-ounce glass of red wine has 128 calories, and a 12-ounce beer packs in 150 calories.

4. Want the heart benefits of red wine without the buzz?
Best drink: purple grape juice.

According to researchers from Georgetown University Medical Center, the flavonoids in red wine—which reduce your blood's stickiness and tendency to clot—are also present in purple grape juice. Other research has shown that purple grape juice helps widen arteries and slow down the speed at which "bad" LDL cholesterol enters the arteries. Read the label, though. You want only 100 percent grape juice (grape juice already has about 40 grams of naturally occurring fructose and glucose, so it's important to avoid any added sugar).

Five More Must-Dos for
Your Best Body

For optimum health, be sure to follow these no-brainer tips as well.

Drink more water. If you take just one lesson away from this chapter (and, of course, I hope you take many more), it's to drink lots of water! My clients swear that getting adequate water changes the quality of their lives. They feel so much more energetic. They go to the bathroom regularly. And their skin glows! Water also helps regulate body temperature. Think hot flashes! A cold glass of water can cool you down from the inside out in about sixty seconds. In fact, most menopausal symptoms, including headaches, mood swings, joint pain, and bloating, can be minimized if you stay hydrated. Remember: your body's thirst mechanism becomes less reliable as you age, so don't wait until you're feeling parched to drink up. Instead, keep the fluids flowing throughout the day.

Kick the caffeine habit. Sleep deprivation and fatigue may make you want to down a double espresso for a quick energy boost. But there can be downsides to caffeine. Even small amounts can make you anxious and jittery or interfere with your sleep. Caffeine also can cause dehydration and breast tenderness. Not to mention that your favorite piping hot latte could bring on a hot flash! If you must have your daily fix, try something decaf and iced.

Keep tabs on your cocktails. In addition to triggering hot flashes, alcohol can deplete the calcium in our bones, setting the stage for osteoporosis. But that doesn't mean you must become a teeto-taler. In moderation, wine and other alcoholic beverages can be "heart smart," as they can raise levels of HDL or "good" choles-terol and may lower blood pressure. Having more than seven drinks a week, however, can increase your risk of heart attack, stroke, and possibly even breast cancer. Besides, those alcohol calo-ries can really add up. Research shows that a pre-dinner cocktail won't keep you from eating less; if anything, it'll make you more apt to overindulge.

Pop a multivitamin. While you can get all the nutrients you need from a healthy and varied diet, most nutrition experts recommend taking a multivitamin just to be safe. Keep in mind that after menopause, your multivitamin doesn't need to contain as much iron—only about 8 milligrams instead of 18. Why? Once your pe-riod stops, you no longer lose iron through menstrual bleeding.

Say "Sayonara" to salt. Not only does excess sodium raise blood pressure, it can cause water retention and contribute to osteo-porosis. Once you hit your forties, the government recommends limiting sodium intake to 1,500 milligrams a day. My advice? Avoid high-sodium foods, such as packaged snacks, salad dressings, jarred sauces, canned soups, and frozen dinners. And chuck your salt shaker! One teaspoon of table salt contains almost 2,300 milligrams of sodium. If you need more flavor, experiment with flavorful, salt-free alternatives, such as garlic, herbs, spices, and lemon.

The Sunday Setup

For many of my clients, the biggest obstacle to healthy eating is convenience. So I often remind them to keep their kitchens stocked with nutritious, easy-to-grab nibbles. The Sunday Setup is how I make it happen. Every Sunday, I go to the grocery store and do my shopping for the week. I plan my weekly menu, check my staples, and make a shopping list. I buy everything I will need, including fruits, vegetables, lean protein, and whole grains such as whole wheat pasta and brown rice. When I get home from the store, I try to spend a few minutes preparing healthy snacks and meals for the coming days. Here are a few of my favorite moves:

- Chop carrots and celery into small sticks. Place them in a glass bowl, add water, and keep them covered and refrigerated.

- Rinse cherry tomatoes and radishes and put them in your prettiest bowl.

- Cut up fresh fruit, such as melon, pineapple, and mango, into chunks and place it in a covered Tupperware container so you can see it clearly.

- Wash a few apples and place them in a bowl near your car keys, so you can grab one on your way out the door.

- Rinse strawberries and arrange them on a plate. I leave on the green, leafy stems because it keeps them fresher longer and makes them look so beautiful.

- Keep a bag of prewashed spinach on hand for superquick salads. I also like adding a handful of spinach leaves to sandwiches, scrambled eggs, and canned soups. It's delicious, nutritious, and easy!

- Wash and bake sweet potatoes and store them in an airtight container in your fridge. (They keep well for about three or four days.) A great source of fiber and beta-carotene, they make an incredibly tasty and satisfying snack.

- Hard-boil eggs and store them in the refrigerator. Slice them up onto salads or eat one whenever you want a protein pick-me-up!

- Grill, roast, or boil chicken breasts for use in sandwiches and salads.

- Cut up bell peppers, zucchini, yellow squash, onions, and eggplant, toss with a little olive oil, and season with just a little salt and pepper. Put them on a baking sheet lined with nonstick foil and roast for 20 to 30 minutes at 400°F. Once cool, store them in the refrigerator. You can add them to salads or toss them with whole wheat pasta for a quick, nutritious meal.

Six Nutrients You Need *Now*

Anthocyanins. These powerful antioxidants have pigments that give certain fruits, vegetables, and other plants their deep purple or purple-red color. They can prevent blood clotting and can inhibit LDL or "bad" cholesterol. They may even lower blood sugar levels and help individuals with diabetes boost their insulin production. Some research also suggests that anthocyanins may reduce pain by minimizing inflammation. Pick up eggplant, black beans, beets, cherries, and blackberries to add this nutritional powerhouse to your diet.

Folate. Also known as folic acid, this B vitamin helps build and maintain new cells. It also helps lower levels of homocysteine in the blood, which is shown to reduce the risk of heart disease and stroke. Consuming foods rich in folate, some studies conclude, also may reduce breast and colon cancer risk. Some research even suggests a link between a lack of dietary folic acid and depression. Citrus fruits, turkey, asparagus, tomatoes, dried beans and peas, and dark, leafy vegetables are all good sources. And some breakfast cereals are fortified with folic acid.

Lutein. In a class of nutrients known as carotenoids, lutein may help prevent atherosclerosis (fatty deposits in blood vessels) as well as macular degeneration, the most common cause of blindness in the elderly. Some scientists consider it as potent as beta-carotene, with the same disease-fighting properties. It can be found in dark, leafy vegetables (such as spinach, kale, and turnip greens), egg yolks, and avocados.

Lycopene. This so-called phytochemical is found in red-hued fruits and vegetables, including tomatoes, watermelon, pink grapefruit, and papaya. It has been linked to a lower risk of prostate, lung, and colon cancer as well as cardiovascular disease. The best sources are cooked or processed tomato products, such as tomato sauce, tomato juice, and tomato soup, and watermelon.   (continued)

Omega-3 fatty acids. Omega-3s are a form of polyunsaturated fats found mainly in cold-water fish—such as salmon, tuna, halibut, and mackerel—that have been shown to help stabilize an irregular heartbeat, lower cholesterol and triglyceride levels, and decrease blood pressure. Some research suggests that they may help reduce the risk of diabetes, ease joint pain, improve memory, and combat depression. To get your fill, the American Heart Association recommends putting the catch of the day on your plate at least twice a week. Other food sources include canola oil, flaxseed, flaxseed oil, walnuts, and leafy greens.

Vitamin E. Another key antioxidant, vitamin E helps protect cells from the damaging effects of free radicals. Some evidence shows that vitamin E can help prevent blocked arteries and blood clots to lower your risk of heart attack. Some studies have shown that increased consumption of vitamin E may decrease the risk of breast cancer (although this finding was inconclusive in one study of postmenopausal women). In the grocery store, you can find vitamin E in most nuts (including walnuts and almonds), soybeans, sunflower seeds, and vegetable oils.

Simply Delicious Recipes

When I put together these recipes for you, not only did I tap into my personal collection, I reached out to my good friend Gavan Murphy. Gavan began his culinary career in Ireland in 1992 and worked his way around the British Isles before arriving in California in 2000. The health-conscious California culture allowed Gavan to combine his interest in exercise, health, and nutrition with his cooking. After working for a number of prestigious Los Angeles catering companies, Gavan took his skills "private," becoming a personal chef as well as a food consultant to a multinational sports nutrition company.

What I love about Gavan (aside from his fabulous recipes!) is that he shares my own eating philosophy: The best way to achieve a fit body is to fuel it with wholesome, nutritious foods. The key word here is *fuel*. Good food keeps our bodies moving and our metabolisms in overdrive, which we need to burn off excess body fat. Like me, Gavan doesn't use the word *diet* in terms of losing weight; to him, it is a lifestyle that involves consuming a variety of nutrient-rich foods from different food groups and enjoying every bite!

The following recipes are designed to introduce you to this world of delicious, healthy eating. Some are quick fixes for one. Others are for your whole family. All of them include important nutrients that will help you fend off those ravages of aging and feel your very best. I hope you love them as much as I do!

Breakfasts

. . . .

Energizing Oatmeal

Whenever I sit down to this high-fiber breakfast, I feel satisfied and energized for hours. Prepare the oatmeal with nonfat milk, or sip a decaf latte for a protein boost. • *Serves 1*

1 cup dry oatmeal

Nonfat milk or water

2 teaspoons dried cranberries or dried plums

2 teaspoons chopped pecans

Prepare oatmeal according to the package directions, using nonfat milk or water. Top with dried fruit and pecans.

Kathy's Favorite Breakfast Burrito

Thanks to the whole wheat tortilla, this supereasy wrap is packed with both protein and fiber. • *Serves 1*

1 whole wheat, burrito-size tortilla

3 egg whites

1 slice nonfat cheese, diced

1 tablespoon salsa

Heat the tortilla in a dry pan over medium heat until lightly browned. Remove and place on a paper towel. In the same pan, scramble the egg whites with the cheese. Spoon the scrambled eggs and cheese along the center of the tortilla and top with salsa. Fold the sides in over the filling, then roll up the tortilla to enclose the filling.

Whole Wheat French Toast

For a little texture, try using a grainy bread, such as Oroweat's Master's Best Winter Wheat, which contains cracked wheat, sunflower seeds, and walnuts. • *Serves 1*

> **1 egg white, beaten with 1 tablespoon nonfat milk**
> **Pinch of cinnamon**
> **Drop of vanilla extract**
> **2 slices whole wheat bread**
> **Mazola Pure cooking spray**
> **1/3 cup fresh raspberries**

In a bowl, beat the egg white with the cinnamon and vanilla. Soak the bread in the egg white mixture. Coat a medium nonstick skillet with cooking spray, then place the bread in the skillet. Cook the egg-soaked bread over medium heat until lightly browned on each side. Top with fresh raspberries.

Fresh Fruit Smoothie

I make this delicious calcium- and protein-packed smoothie all the time. It's great first thing in the morning or as a post-workout refresher. • *Serves 1*

> **1 cup unsweetened frozen strawberries**
> **1 medium banana**
> **1/4 cup frozen blueberries**
> **1/2 cup nonfat milk**
> **2 tablespoons protein powder**

Combine all ingredients in a blender. Blend on high speed until smooth and creamy.

Whole-Grain Cranberry Nut Muffin

I used to think of muffins as a no-no. Then I discovered this healthy recipe. It's so good that you'll be fighting your kids for seconds! • *Serves 12*

1½ cups whole wheat flour

¾ cup quick-cooking oats

⅔ cup light brown sugar

2 teaspoons baking powder

¼ teaspoon salt

1 cup fresh or frozen cranberries, chopped

½ cup chopped pecans or almonds

1 tablespoon orange zest (finely grated orange peel)

2 large eggs

¾ cup nonfat or low-fat milk

⅓ cup canola oil

½ teaspoon vanilla extract

Preheat the oven to 350°F. In a medium bowl, mix the flour, oats, sugar, baking powder, and salt, then stir in the cranberries and nuts. In a small bowl, mix the orange zest, eggs, milk, oil, and vanilla. Add the wet ingredients to the dry ingredients, stirring until blended (don't beat the batter; it will make the muffins tough). Fill 12 paper-lined muffin cups about three-quarters full. Bake for 18 to 20 minutes, or until golden brown. Remove from the oven. Let cool for at least 5 minutes before digging in.

Lunches

. . . .

Vegetarian Chili

Whip up this easy chili on Sunday, and you'll have healthy lunches for the next several days. The tomatoes are a great source of the antioxidant lycopene, while the beans provide protein and fiber. • *Serves 4*

- **1 medium onion, chopped**
- **2 garlic cloves, chopped**
- **1 green bell pepper, chopped**
- **1 tablespoon olive oil**
- **2 tablespoons chili powder**
- **One 15-ounce can red kidney beans, drained**
- **One 15-ounce can crushed tomatoes**

In a medium saucepan over medium heat, sauté the onion, garlic, and pepper in the oil until soft. Add the chili powder, beans, and tomatoes. Cover and cook over medium heat for 1 hour. Spoon into your favorite chili bowl and enjoy!

Ginger Lime Shrimp Salad

This light, luscious salad from Gavan Murphy is one of my new lunch favorites. • *Serves 2*

SHRIMP MARINADE

1 tablespoon grated fresh ginger

Zest and juice of 1 lime

Pinch of cayenne pepper

ASIAN VINAIGRETTE

2 tablespoons rice vinegar

$1/4$ cup soy sauce

1 tablespoon honey

SHRIMP SALAD

8 ounces tiger shrimp, peeled and deveined

1 cup Napa cabbage, cleaned and shredded

1 cup red cabbage, shredded

1 cup romaine lettuce, chopped

1 tablespoon chopped fresh mint

Salt and pepper

$1/2$ cup red or yellow cherry tomatoes, halved

1 papaya, peeled and diced

To make the marinade, whisk together the marinade ingredients in a medium bowl. Place the shrimp in the bowl, cover, and marinate in the fridge for 1 hour. To make the vinaigrette, whisk together the vinaigrette ingredients. Mix the Napa and red cabbages, romaine lettuce, and mint together and drizzle with some of the vinaigrette to coat. Season lightly with salt and pepper. In a medium-hot pan, sauté the shrimp for 2 minutes on each side. Season lightly with salt and pepper. Divide the green salad between 2 plates and sprinkle each with the tomatoes and papaya. Arrange the shrimp on each.

Chopped Vegetable Salad

This antioxidant-packed salad really couldn't be any simpler!

• *Serves 2*

1 cucumber, peeled and chopped

1 red bell pepper, diced

3 celery stalks, diced

1 cup cherry tomatoes, halved

2 tablespoons chopped red onion

1 tablespoon lime juice

Combine all ingredients and serve.

Niçoise Salad with Seared Ahi

I don't know how a chef from Ireland learned to make Niçoise Salad—but it's amazing, and loaded with good-for-you ingredients!

• *Serves* 2

8 ounces fresh ahi, or albacore tuna in water

Salt and pepper

4 cups mixed salad greens

½ cup plum tomatoes, diced into large pieces

½ cup peeled and diced cucumber

8 ounces (1 handful) fresh green beans, blanched and
    refreshed in ice water

¼ cup pitted black olives, halved

1 cup cooked new potatoes, halved

2 large hard-boiled eggs, cut into quarters

Lemon wedges, optional

VINAIGRETTE

2 tablespoons olive oil

½ teaspoon whole-grain mustard

1 tablespoon balsamic vinegar

Salt and pepper

Season all sides of the ahi with salt and pepper to taste. Heat a skillet on high heat, add the ahi, and sear on all sides for 30 seconds only, so as not to overcook. Remove the ahi from the heat and let stand at room temperature. To make the vinaigrette, whisk together the vinaigrette ingredients. Mix the greens, tomatoes, cucumber, beans, olives, and potatoes and toss in enough vinaigrette to coat. Season with salt and pepper to taste. Divide the tossed salad between 2 plates. Gently lay egg quarters around the sides of each plate. Once the ahi has cooled, slice it thinly and arrange on top of the salad. Drizzle the remaining vinaigrette over the ahi and serve with lemon wedges, if using. *Bon appétit!*

Homemade Turkey Burger
with Asian Slaw

You may never go back to hamburgers once you've had one of
Gavan's tasty, low-fat turkey burgers. • *Serves 2*

1 tablespoon olive oil

1 small red onion, finely diced

1 garlic clove, minced

8 ounces ground white turkey meat

1 tablespoon whole-grain mustard

1 tablespoon chopped fresh tarragon

1 tablespoon Worcestershire sauce

Salt and pepper

2 cups shredded cabbage
   (prepackaged in most stores)

2 whole wheat burger buns

Lettuce and sliced tomatoes, optional

VINAIGRETTE

$1/2$ tablespoon rice vinegar

1 tablespoon honey

1 teaspoon Dijon mustard

Soy sauce

1 tablespoon sesame oil

Salt and pepper

Heat the olive oil in a medium pan, then sauté the onion on medium
heat for about 5 minutes. Add the garlic and reduce the heat. Cook
the onion and garlic until translucent. Set aside. Mix the turkey,
mustard, tarragon, Worcestershire sauce, and cooled onion mixture.
Season with salt and pepper to taste. If you like, cook a small portion
of the turkey to make sure you like the seasoning. When you're
satisfied, make two burgers. Grill or broil the burgers. To make the

vinaigrette, mix the vinegar, honey, mustard, and a drizzle of soy sauce. Whisk in the sesame oil and season with salt and pepper to taste. Toss the slaw mix with the vinaigrette. Serve the cooked burgers on the buns, with the slaw on the side. Top the burgers with lettuce and tomato, if using.

Snacks

· · · · · · · · · · ·

Fresh Cut Garden Veggies with Apple Mint Yogurt Dip

When Gavan first introduced me to this dip, I was skeptical. Apple and mint? Now I can't get enough of it! It's a simple and nutritious snack that can be kept in the fridge for an anytime snack. Cut up the veggies and keep them in airtight containers in the fridge for quick snacking.

Carrots

Celery

Cucumber

Green beans, blanched

Snow peas, blanched

Broccoli, blanched

Asparagus, blanched

Cherry tomatoes

Bell peppers (green, yellow, red, or orange)

DIP

1 apple (any variety), chopped

¼ cup fresh mint

8 ounces yogurt, low-fat or nonfat, any flavor

To make the dip, mix the apple, mint, and yogurt. Chill. Dip the veggies when you need a quick snack!

Homemade Tomato and Avocado Dip with Pita Chips

You don't need to wait for your next party to enjoy this healthy dip from Gavan Murphy. Instead celebrate all the healthy benefits of avocado, including its artery-loving monounsaturated fat and powerful antioxidant, glutathione. • *Serves 2*

DIP

2 plum tomatoes, finely diced

1 avocado, finely diced

1 teaspoon finely diced red onion

Zest and juice of 1 lime

1 teaspoon chopped fresh cilantro

Salt and pepper

PITA CHIPS

2 whole wheat pita pockets

Pinch of cayenne pepper

Olive oil

Dash of salt

Preheat the oven to 350°F. Gently mix the tomatoes, avocado, onion, lime zest and juice, cilantro, and salt and pepper to taste. Chill. To make the pita chips, cut the pita pockets into 8 pieces each. In a small bowl mix the cayenne, oil, and salt. Toss the pita pieces in this mixture. Place the pita pieces on a cookie sheet and bake for 15 minutes. Cool the pita pieces, break out the dip, and serve.

Grilled Chicken 'n' Onion Pizza

Gavan's protein-packed mini-pizza is perfect as an afternoon snack or a light lunch. You can prepare the chicken ahead of time, or use leftover chicken from a previous meal. • *Serves 2*

1 tablespoon olive oil

1 medium red onion, thinly sliced

1 garlic clove, minced

2 chicken breasts, 4 ounces each

4 tablespoons pizza or marinara sauce

2 whole wheat pita pockets

1 teaspoon chopped fresh thyme

2 tablespoons low-fat Jack, Cheddar, or American cheese

Freshly ground black pepper

Preheat the oven to 350°F. Heat the oil in a medium pan, then sauté the onion and garlic on medium-low heat for 15 to 20 minutes, until the mixture begins to caramelize. Season and grill the chicken. Slice the chicken. To assemble the pizzas, spread the pizza sauce on each pita pocket. Arrange the chicken, onion mixture, and cheese on top of the sauce. Sprinkle with pepper and thyme to taste. Bake for 5 to 10 minutes. Do not overbake, as the pita bread will continue to crisp once it is out of the oven.

Zucchini-Jicama Dip with Fresh Veggies

If you've never tried jicama, prepare to fall in love with its crisp, cool flavor • *Serves 4*

1 cup shredded zucchini

1 cup shredded jicama

2 garlic cloves, crushed

Pinch of salt and pepper

1/2 cup plain nonfat or low-fat yogurt

Fresh veggies, cleaned and cut for dipping

Combine the zucchini, jicama, garlic, salt, and pepper in a small bowl and stir well. Let the mixture stand for at least 30 minutes at room temperature. Press the mixture between paper towels to remove excess moisture. Combine the zucchini mixture and the yogurt, stirring well. Cover and chill. Serve with fresh raw veggies.

Kathy's Popcorn

This healthy snack is low in calories and filled with fiber.

For the best popcorn, skip the microwave and get a Whirley Pop Popcorn Popper. I got mine a few years ago at Williams-Sonoma, but you can also order one online at www.popcornpopper.com. All you need is your favorite popcorn and a tiny bit of olive oil. I like using Baby White Gourmet Popcorn from www.givemepopcorn.com. To jazz it up, add a few shakes of Parmesan cheese right after you put the popcorn in the bowl. Movie, anyone?

Spicy Pepitas

Sometimes we all need a little crunch. So why not crunch healthy? Pumpkin seeds are packed with nutrients and, when "spiced up," make a terrific snack. • *Serves 6–8*

> **3 tablespoons freshly squeezed lime juice**
>
> **$1/4$ teaspoon black pepper**
>
> **$1/4$ teaspoon cayenne pepper**
>
> **$1/2$ teaspoon salt**
>
> **$1^{1}/_{2}$ to 2 cups pepitas (raw hulled green pumpkin seeds)**

Mix the lime juice, black pepper, cayenne, and salt. Stir until the seasonings dissolve. Heat a large skillet over medium heat. Add the pepitas and toss frequently until they begin to turn golden brown. Add the seasoned lime juice and stir well until all the pepitas are coated. Remove from the heat and cool in the pan. Serve these healthy and delicious seeds at room temperature.

Dinners

. . . .

Broccoli and Tofu Stir-Fry

Tofu is a great addition to your diet. It's loaded with protein and calcium, and is a terrific change from chicken! If you make the rice ahead of time, you can have a tasty, nutritious dinner on the table in less than ten minutes. • *Serves 2*

> 2 garlic cloves, chopped
>
> 2 cups broccoli florets
>
> 4 ounces baked sesame or teriyaki seasoned tofu,
> cut into $1/4$-inch cubes
>
> 3 tablespoons low-sodium soy sauce
>
> 1 cup cooked brown rice

Heat the garlic over medium heat in a medium nonstick saucepan. Once the garlic begins to brown, toss in the broccoli. When the broccoli turns bright green, add the tofu. Cook another 3 minutes, stirring occasionally. Add the soy sauce, and cook another minute. Serve over the brown rice.

Turkey Meat Loaf

Everyone in my house likes this healthy, lower-fat twist on traditional meat loaf. • *Serves 4*

1 garlic clove, crushed

2 tablespoons chopped onion

1 teaspoon olive oil

1 pound ground, low-fat turkey breast

$1/2$ cup nonfat marinara sauce

$1/2$ cup bread crumbs

$1/2$ cup dry instant oats

1 egg white, beaten

2 teaspoons chopped fresh parsley

Additional $1/4$ cup marinara sauce to top meat loaf

Preheat the oven to 350°F. In a small saucepan over medium heat, lightly sauté the garlic and onion in the oil. Combine the garlic mixture with the turkey, marinara sauce, bread crumbs, oats, egg white, and parsley. Mix thoroughly and pack into a 4 x 9-inch loaf pan. Top with the additional marinara sauce and bake for 40 minutes. Comfort food at its best!

Herb-Roasted Turkey Breast

A three-pound turkey breast will make four generous servings, plus provide plenty of leftovers for hearty sandwiches. • *Serves 4*

1 boneless rolled turkey breast (3 pounds)

1 teaspoon olive oil

1 teaspoon dried rosemary

2 teaspoons ground thyme

1 teaspoon freshly ground black pepper

2 large sweet potatoes, diced

2 medium white onions, peeled and quartered

Preheat the oven to 375°F. Rub the turkey breast with the oil, rosemary, thyme, and pepper. Place in a medium baking pan, surrounded by the potatoes and onions. Roast for 1^1/$_2$ hours, turning the vegetables occasionally to brown evenly. Remove from the oven, allowing the turkey to rest on a platter for 10 minutes before carving. Serve with the roasted potatoes and onions for an everyday Thanksgiving.

Cajun Salmon Salad with Arugula Mixed Greens

Looking for a dinner that's packed with taste and nutrients? Look no further. Gavan has created a salad that's rich in omega-3s, vitamins A and C, and folate. • *Serves 2*

12 ounces trimmed asparagus

Zest of 1 lemon

Salt and pepper

1 tablespoon olive oil

2 salmon pieces, 6 ounces each

½ teaspoon Cajun seasoning

4 cups arugula mixed greens

½ cup red or yellow cherry tomatoes, halved

4 tablespoons reduced-fat blue cheese

Lemon wedges, optional

VINAIGRETTE

Zest and juice of 1 lemon

2 tablespoons olive oil

1 teaspoon chopped chives or green onion

Salt and pepper

Preheat the oven to 350°F. Toss the asparagus with the lemon zest, salt and pepper to taste, and oil. Then roast for 20 to 25 minutes, until tender. Coat the top side of each salmon piece with the Cajun seasoning. Grill the salmon until cooked through. Divide the greens between 2 plates, topping with the asparagus and tomatoes. To make the vinaigrette, mix the lemon zest and juice, oil, chives, and salt and pepper to taste. Drizzle the vinaigrette over the greens and sprinkle with the blue cheese. Add the salmon. Serve with lemon wedges, if using.

Spinach Salad with Almond Chicken

Combine healthy almonds with nutrient-rich spinach, and you've got a winning combination for your heart and your taste buds. • *Serves 2*

2 tablespoons balsamic vinegar

2 tablespoons olive oil

$\frac{1}{4}$ teaspoon freshly ground black pepper

1 boneless, skinless chicken breast (5 ounces)

1 tablespoon cornstarch

2 egg whites, or $\frac{1}{4}$ cup liquid egg substitute

1 tablespoon finely chopped almonds

3 cups fresh spinach leaves

$\frac{1}{4}$ cup sliced mushrooms

$\frac{1}{2}$ cup yellow and red grape tomatoes, cut in half

In a medium bowl, whisk together the vinegar, 1 tablespoon of the oil, and the pepper. Let stand. Sprinkle each side of the chicken breast with the cornstarch. Dip the chicken into the egg whites to coat and then sprinkle with the almonds. Coat a medium skillet with the remaining olive oil and heat over medium heat. Sauté the chicken for 5 minutes on each side, or until cooked through. Place the chicken on a cutting board to cool slightly. Whisk the dressing again. Add the spinach and toss, then add the mushrooms and tomatoes. Slice the chicken diagonally and place on top of the salad. Enjoy!

Spicy Cajun Crispy Chicken

I make this incredibly easy dish for my boys all the time, and it's always a hit! It's a great recipe to put together in the morning before you leave for work or after the kids are off to school. • *Serves 4*

> **4 skinless chicken breasts (4 to 5 ounces each)**
> **³/₄ cup nonfat yogurt**
> **2¹/₂ cups Total cereal**
> **2 teaspoons ground paprika**
> **2 teaspoons Cajun seasoning**
> **Mazola Pure cooking spray**

Preheat the oven to 400°F. Coat the chicken breasts with the yogurt. Refrigerate for a few hours or overnight. Place the cereal in a blender and process into crumbs. Combine the cereal crumbs, paprika, and Cajun seasoning in a small resealable bag and mix. Individually place each chicken breast in the seasoning bag and shake to coat evenly. Place the seasoned chicken breasts on a baking sheet lightly coated with cooking spray and bake for 40 to 50 minutes, or until done.

Side Dishes

Grilled Zucchini

Pair this side dish with roasted salmon or turkey meat loaf for a delicious dose of potassium, folate, and vitamin A. • *Serves 2*

1 garlic clove, crushed

1 teaspoon olive oil

2 medium zucchini, sliced thinly lengthwise

Preheat a ridged grill pan over high heat until very hot. Stir the garlic into the oil in a small bowl. Lightly brush the zucchini slices with the garlic-flavored oil and grill for about 2 minutes on each side, until you see brown grill lines on the surface. For the best flavor texture, allow the grilled zucchini to rest for 30 minutes before enjoying, but if time is short, it will still taste great hot off the grill!

Baked Fries

Let's face it. We all love French fries. So I've created a healthy alternative that will satisfy your craving (it works for me!). If you want to add an extra antioxidant punch, try using sweet potatoes or a combination of sweet and regular potatoes. • *Serves 4*

3 large baking potatoes

1 egg white

2 teaspoons ground paprika

2 teaspoons garlic powder

1/2 teaspoon seasoned salt

1/2 teaspoon freshly ground black pepper

Mazola Pure cooking spray

Preheat the oven to 400°F. Clean the potatoes and cut into 1/4- to 1/2-inch strips. Pat the potatoes dry with a paper towel and place them in a bowl. Add the egg white and spices and mix, tossing to coat evenly. Spray a baking sheet with cooking spray and spread the potatoes in a single layer across the pan. Bake for 30 minutes, or until golden brown. This is one of my absolute favorites!

Smashed Potatoes

Creamy mashed potatoes don't have to be a thing of the past. Instead of using heavy cream and sticks of butter, follow my recipe for a healthy alternative. • *Serves 4*

1½ pounds red-skinned new potatoes, peeled and cut
    into 1-inch pieces

3 tablespoons nonfat milk

1 tablespoon butter

2½ tablespoons finely chopped fresh basil

1 tablespoon Parmesan, grated

1 teaspoon minced garlic

Salt and pepper

Bring a pot of salted water to a boil. Add the potatoes and cook until tender. Drain the potatoes. Combine the milk and butter in a small saucepan and heat until the butter melts. Transfer the potatoes to a medium mixing bowl. Add the milk mixture, basil, Parmesan, and garlic. Beat with an electric mixer until fluffy. Season with salt and pepper to taste. You won't want to go back to your grandmother's recipe!

Drinks

. . . .

Cucumber-Mint Water

If you've ever been to a day spa, chances are you've tried cucumber water. It's refreshing and rejuvenating. It's a great alternative to diet soda or mineral water.

> **2 quarts cold water**
> **1 seedless cucumber, thinly sliced**
> **¼ cup fresh mint leaves**

Put the cucumber and mint in a large pitcher. Using a wooden spoon, blend the ingredients and press them together. Add 2 quarts cold water and steep for 30 minutes. Using a small strainer, pour the water into another pitcher filled with ice. Enjoy before, during, and after your workout.

Lemon-Mint Ice Cubes

For a special treat, add some flavored ice cubes to your water or seltzer.

> **1½ cups water**
> **½ cup fresh lemon juice**
> **2 tablespoons sugar**
> **Mint leaves for each ice cube section**

Combine the water, lemon juice, and sugar in a small bowl. Stir until the sugar dissolves. Pour the mixture into a standard ice cube tray. Add 1 mint leaf to each cube and freeze.

Raspberry Wonder

This is a great post-workout drink! • *Serves 1–2*

1 cup frozen raspberries

3 ounces silken soft tofu

**1 cup orange juice (to add more calcium to your diet,
use calcium-fortified OJ)**

½ banana

Combine all ingredients in a blender. Blend until smooth. Pour into glasses and drink immediately.

Lemon Sparkler

Looking for something other than plain lemon water? Try this for yourself or make some for friends for an afternoon refresher.

6 lemon herbal tea bags

Sparkling water

Lemon wedges

Boil 2 cups water. Place the tea bags in a teapot, pour the boiling water over them, and steep for 5 minutes. Remove the bags and chill. When ready to serve, fill a glass with half lemon tea and half sparkling water. Garnish with a lemon wedge and enjoy!

5

. . . .

It's a New Chapter
of Our Lives

Let's Make It a Page-Turner!

A FEW DECADES AGO, menopause was rarely discussed. Many of our mothers went through the passage without acknowledging it, even to their closest friends and confidantes. All we heard were hushed references to "the change," if it was mentioned at all. Why were women covering up this inherently natural part of being female? Because of embarrassment, the hesitation to discuss "womanly issues," or a general lack of understanding of what was happening to them?

Since then, we've come a long way. Menopause is now talked about openly in magazines and on the news, and we have much more information on how to stay healthy and deal with the symptoms. Still, for some of you, menopause remains a private matter, and not something that you want to advertise to the world. I suspect part of it may have to do with getting older. Despite all the sexy images we see of women in their forties and fifties these days—on magazine covers, movie and television screens, and the like—there's still somewhat of a stigma about aging. And yes, it *can* have a negative impact on our careers, our desirability, and our feelings about ourselves . . . but *only* if we let it!

. . . .

"There are some positives that come with aging. For one, I feel much more comfortable in my skin. I don't have to worry about impressing people anymore. I don't feel like I need to change to please anyone. I've accepted myself the way I am. And you know what? I'm a pretty damn decent person."

—Marsha, age sixty-two

. . . .

I'll confess: Before signing up to write a book on aging and menopause, I had to think twice. Did I really want tens of thousands of people knowing my age and intimate details about my body and other parts of my life? But ultimately, I decided that a lot of good could come from opening up about it—for all of us. And I was right, at least as far as I'm concerned. This book has inspired me to communicate with my family and friends, explore my feelings, learn about the different treatment options, and approach getting older with a sense of optimism.

In my research, I discovered that the transitional phase of perimenopause can be referred to as *climacteric*. There are several definitions of *climacteric*, but my favorite is "a critical period in a person's life when major changes in health or fortune are thought to take place." Notice that the definition refers to a person, not just a woman, because everyone changes and grows older. And it's not the end of something but a direct link between change and fortune.

In my book (literally!), this new phase isn't viewed as an ending. Really, it's the beginning of countless opportunities to embrace change and to find the fortune in that change. While we may be closing one chapter of our lives, we're starting a new one filled with promise and possibilities. So no more hushed voices. Let's stop thinking of it as something to be ashamed of and enduring it in silence. Instead, let's start challenging the negative stereotypes and expressing our emotions to our partners, our families, and our friends. We're women, we're fabulous, and we're embracing and loving our new selves. And we're starting now.

Of course, I realize it's not always easy to be positive, especially when your hormones are raging and you don't know how you'll feel from one moment to the next. That's what this chapter is for—to help you navigate this crazy midlife adventure and to be your healthiest, happiest, most beautiful self. There will be obstacles along the way, but following my tips and suggestions will help you overcome each challenge and keep your vitality and sanity in the days and years to come.

Accept Your Body

As I've already told you, I've struggled with body image issues much of my life. While some of this struggle was about control issues, it was also triggered by my desire to have a certain body type—one that I wasn't born with. I wasn't overweight, but I thought I was too fat at the time.

Now that I'm in my midforties, and I'm gaining weight and getting thicker around the middle, I would love to have my old body back. Oh, the irony! Now, when I look back at old photographs from, say, college or my wedding day, I think I looked fantastic. Why couldn't I see it at the time? Why didn't I always treat my body with the respect it deserved? At this point, I've realized that I'm never going to completely love my body. But I've learned to accept and appreciate it. And I've learned to stop comparing myself to others—especially women with different bone structures and those younger than I am. And so can you.

Which brings me to another point. Some of you may have young daughters who are starting to blossom. Daughters who are getting their periods for the first time. Daughters who can eat anything they want and still look great in a bikini. If you don't have a daughter, maybe you have a teenage son who is dating some pretty young thing. (It's not too far away for me with my three sons!) If you think back long and hard enough, you may actually remember when you looked that way.

. . . .

"We guys are really ignorami on this 'taboo' topic. If women don't understand completely what is happening and are not prone to discuss it, even among themselves, husbands who may wish to be supportive of their wives are left even more in the dark."

—Ned, age sixty

. . . .

If there's one thing that I've learned from living in Los Angeles—and training incredibly beautiful women such as Julia Roberts, Jennifer Aniston, Michelle Pfeiffer, and Cindy Crawford for a living—it's to avoid trying to be something that I'm not. I'm not twenty anymore, so I can't expect to look like a twenty-year-old. Instead, I'm going to work hard to make my forty-four-year-old body the best that it can be.

When it comes to our figures, it's important to recognize that some things are within our control, and others aren't. At five feet, seven inches tall, I weigh more than 150 pounds. I'm strong and muscular. I have big bones. Sure, I could stand to lose a few pounds, but I'll never have a super-skinny body. I'll never have abs like Jennifer Aniston, especially after having three babies. I'll never have Cindy Crawford's long legs or Julia Roberts's slender arms. It's just not in my genetic cards. What can I do except get over it? *Let it go. Let it go. Let it go.*

No one likes wrinkles, but when you think about it, a face with lines has much more depth and character than a face without lines. After all, those lines tell a story. One may tell a tale of heartbreak. The ex-boyfriend who dumped you. The dream job that you didn't get. The death of a loved one. Another may tell a tale of happiness. The day you got married. The birth of a child. Your very first kiss.

A few years ago, actress Jamie Lee Curtis posed in nothing more than a jog bra and spandex briefs for *More* magazine. Many of us were shocked to see the then forty-three-year-old—who is known for her incredibly lean, sexy figure—looking, well, like the rest of us. She agreed to do the photo shoot because she wanted other women in their forties to know the truth. As she put it, "I don't have great thighs. I have very big breasts and a soft, fatty little tummy. And I've got back fat. People assume that I'm walking around in little spaghetti-strap dresses . . . I don't want the unsuspecting forty-year-old women of the world to think that I've got it going on. It's such a fraud. And I'm the one perpetuating it."

In the same article, Jamie Lee admitted having had plastic surgery years earlier. But now, what she really wants is to feel at peace with her flaws. I felt so good after reading her story. It really reinforced that we don't have to be perfect. It's just the media that makes us feel that way.

Emphasize the Positives

It's unfortunate, but as women, we're often gifted at seeing the good in others but unable to focus on our own positive traits. Instead of looking in the mirror and seeing a devoted mother, an accomplished businesswoman, or a loving wife, we see chubby thighs, an unsightly blemish (which, trust me, no one else notices), or gray hair. During menopause, these kinds of negative thoughts can drag our already low self-esteem into the basement. Which means that we need to retrain ourselves to focus on our good qualities instead of our perceived inadequacies and failures.

Next time you find yourself obsessing over your love handles, for example, try admiring your Marilyn Monroe curves (did you know she was a size fourteen? Or that Lucille Ball, my favorite actress, was a size twelve?). If you were one of the last people to finish the local walk/run, who cares? You did it! That's what's important. So you're not a CEO or a top muckety-muck at your job. Who needs that extra stress anyway? I'll admit that this isn't easy, and it takes practice. But it's something you need to do for yourself. You have so many good qualities. It's time to appreciate each and every one of them instead of always seeing the negatives.

. . . .

"My advice is, talk to your friends about what you're going through. I have a bunch of close girlfriends that I've known for years and years. They've been my lifeline through this whole thing. Menopause is just a natural part of what we talk about. It was comforting to know that I wasn't the only one having a hard time."

—Mary, age fifty

. . . .

While this may sound a little corny (remember Stuart Smalley from *Saturday Night Live* with his "I'm good enough, I'm smart enough, and doggone it, people like me"?), it's effective. When I'm having an "I hate my whatever" moment, I've learned to focus on something I'm proud of, such as helping one client train so she could take a hiking trip to Canada. Or working with local mothers to improve their health. We're not perfect, true. But why waste our energy (and it *is* a waste of energy!) blaming ourselves for our small imperfections when we can give ourselves a much-deserved moment of appreciation?

Here are a few more examples of how to rewrite the negative scripts that play in our minds as we age. Instead of thinking that you're all washed up, remind yourself that you're older and wiser and more grounded. Instead of worrying that you're no longer the new kid at work with exciting new ideas, take the lead as the seasoned veteran that everyone looks up to. Instead of feeling like you haven't done anything with your life, reflect on all you've accomplished over the years. Instead of dwelling on the fact that you'll never outrun a twenty-something on the tennis court, remember that you have the experience to outsmart her.

Cope with Those Crazy Moods

During perimenopause, the monthly mood swings that we've experienced for decades now feel like full-scale emotional tsunamis. Is it really possible to go from delight to despair in 3.5 seconds flat? You bet.

In Chapter 3, I gave you exercises to help elevate your mood. While physical activity can be extremely helpful, other "sanity savers" can help you keep that emotional roller coaster from turning your world upside down.

1. Take a deep breath. Sure, it sounds cliché, but it really does help. It brings vital oxygen into your body, which helps stabilize your energy and your emotions. *Ahhh . . .*

2. Think before you speak. With three children, I've had those pull-your-hair-out moments. I've learned, though, to assess the situation before reacting. I also think that whatever they're doing right now is the same thing they did yesterday, so I shouldn't take it personally or lash out just because my hormones are raging like a California wildfire.

3. Get connected. Isolation can be dangerous, and can lead to feelings of loneliness and despair. So reach out to others. Spending time with friends can help take your mind off your troubles and give you a sense of belonging. About one evening a month, I get together with a group of friends to play a dice game called Bunko. We bring food and drinks, and usually spend the whole night chatting and laughing. I always feel so elated afterward. Some women I know have started book clubs or planned weekly girls' nights. Others have started carpooling to work. You'd take the time to schedule a formal therapy session, right? Well, call your friends and schedule regular informal sessions. You'll all benefit!

4. *Talk about it!* Whenever I'm going through a challenging time, I find that it really helps to talk it out. A good venting session with a girlfriend always makes me feel a thousand times better. So whenever you're in a rotten mood or feeling down, try calling a friend, preferably one who is also going through a similar time in life. It will give you an opportunity to voice your concerns and have your feelings validated. I also recommend opening up to your family. It's especially important to let your significant other and/or kids know what's going on so you get the support and understanding you need. Our loved ones aren't psychics. They won't know what's upsetting you or why you're so moody if you don't try to explain.

"Dear Diary: I'm Feeling *Very* Hormonal Today . . ."

One of my favorite forms of "therapy" is writing in a journal. Every night before bed, I try to spend five or ten minutes writing about my day's events or whatever happens to be on my mind. It's a "safe" place where I can really explore my emotions and be as open and honest as I want to be. When something's troubling me, it can help me clarify my feelings, blow off steam, and clear my head. And I love looking back periodically and reflecting on where I was then compared with where I am now. Try it and see!

5. *Let yourself grieve.* Maybe some of you never got an opportunity to have the baby that you so desperately wanted; others may have wanted a second or third child, but didn't get a chance. Even though I didn't plan on getting pregnant again, the idea of not having any more children still fills me with sadness. It feels like a door is closing forever. It's normal to have feelings of loss as you traverse through menopause. The best thing to do is to allow yourself to grieve. Don't be afraid to cry or scream at the top of your lungs, if it'll help. You don't want to keep it bottled up. Then start thinking about ways to fill that void in your life, whether it's spending more time with your nieces and nephews, adopting a child, or reaching out to a friend in need. A lot of people in the world need a mother's love. They don't have to come from your own womb.

"If you act as though menopause is shameful, it only makes it worse. Instead, I try to joke about it. For example, I often refer to my expanding waist as a water cooler. Humor is always my way of getting through tough times."

—Rene, age forty-eight

6. *Reach out for help.* If your emotions are extreme, seem uncontrollable, or interfere with your day-to-day functioning, you may be experiencing severe anxiety or clinical depression. Call your physician. Professional assistance is available and may take the form of therapy or medications. For others, relaxation techniques may work. If you have any concerns at all, don't hesitate to contact your caregiver. It's better to ask questions and get help than to suffer unnecessarily.

7. Laugh about it! Humor is an amazing gift. It can defuse a tense situation. It can bring people together. It can simply elevate your mood. Pick up a book by Erma Bombeck—she found every situation in life cause for laughter. Joke with your friends about the changes in your bodies and your moods. Or, if you live in a major city such as Chicago or San Francisco, search online to see if Menopause the Musical is in a theater near you. The comedy revue pokes fun at things such as hot flashes, memory loss, mood swings, and wrinkles.

Say "No" to Stress

Too much to do. Too little time. That essentially sums up the state of my life these days. I have a running joke with my next-door neighbor: Whenever I talk to her, one of us will say, "Have you showered yet today? Have you brushed your teeth yet today?" I'm embarrassed to say that my answer is often "No." Some days, I'm so busy that I feel like there's barely time to sit down.

Truth be told, I like being busy. I actually find that I'm more productive when I'm juggling a lot of different things. It forces me to be more efficient with my time. But sometimes, I do take on too much—and that's when I can run into trouble. There's so much to do that I can't focus on anything. As soon as I start feeling overwhelmed, I start getting bitchy.

Let's face it, many of us have an incredible amount on our plates. As wives, mothers, sisters, daughters, and friends, we have a lot of people to care for. Some of us may be concerned about paying for our children's educations and having money for retirement. Others have aging parents who need our help. Our careers may cause additional stress as we take on more responsibilities, or we're worried about keeping our jobs in light of layoffs, early "retirement" packages, and economic woes. Add to the mix mood swings, sleep deprivation, and low self-esteem, and it's no wonder we often feel frazzled and unable to cope.

While being busy isn't bad, being stressed out is very different. As I explained in Chapter 1, chronic stress can be bad for your health and cause you to pack on excess pounds. But don't worry: I'm not going to tell you to just *relax*. And I won't suggest an afternoon at a day spa or a tropical vacation. Sure, a little downtime can do wonders, but not everyone can afford to spend hours getting rubbed down or jet off to the Turks and Caicos. Plus these kinds of solutions simply put a temporary bandage on your problems. So instead, try these real-life, stress-busting strategies that work for me every day:

1. Get organized. Maybe it's my German blood, but I'm one of those people who need to have everything in its place. I find that I'm much more relaxed when my home and office are organized and tidy. It makes me feel calmer, and I don't waste time or get frustrated looking for things, such as my sunglasses or car keys. I'm also a fanatic list maker. I start each day by making a to-do list. I know exactly what I have to do; I can organize my day by prioritizing tasks, streamlining items, and even delegating a chore or two. If I have to go to the post office and the pharmacy, why make two trips when I can take care of both tasks in the same trip? There is also a certain satisfaction in crossing items off the list. And that feeling of accomplishment, for me, is energizing.

2. Don't get overwhelmed. It's easy to get stressed when you have a gazillion things to do. Instead of getting overwhelmed, break it down into little pieces. In other words, focus on what you need to do today, rather than worrying about tomorrow or next week. Then, take one small task—for example, answering e-mails—and sit down and complete the task before you move on to the next thing. This is where list making can really help. If you go down the list, checking off items one by one, you'll be more efficient and productive, which can help lower stress. If it's a larger project (writing this book, for instance), set small, realistic goals and stick to them. The more you procrastinate, the more it will weigh on your mind.

3. Learn to delegate. From cooking and cleaning to grocery shopping and buying gifts, many of us try to do it all ourselves. Sometimes it's a control thing—we want it done our way. In other instances, it just seems easier than assigning the task to someone else. Or maybe it's just a reluctance to ask for help. I used to be that way. But over the years, I've learned to be a good delegator. Recently I've been producing plays for my children's school. But because of all the things I have going on in my life, I've delegated much of the physical work to other parents. By delegating, you open yourself up to other people's input and ideas, which can result in a better end product. No, they may not do it your way. But you may discover that their method is just as effective—and may even teach you something new.

Part of managing stress is learning to relax. I do several things to find calm in my crazy life:

1. Take up a hobby. Find a hobby that is unrelated to your work, so you can focus on something different. Some of my friends have become regular Martha Stewarts, knitting, crocheting, and scrapbooking their way to stress-free evenings. I like unwinding with Sudoku, the latest puzzle rage. You can find it in the newspaper, usually near the crossword puzzle. There are also lots of Sudoku books on the market. It's a fun, challenging, and addictive grid pattern that takes your mind away from just about everything else.

2. Enjoy a cup of tea. Waiting for the water to boil, brewing a cup of your favorite (decaffeinated!) blend, and sitting down to enjoy a cozy beverage force you to slow down. You don't have to go, go, go every minute of the day. So once in a while, take a break and relax with a soothing cup of chamomile tea.

3. Soothe your baby blues (or greens or browns). With all of the environmental influences irritating our eyes, and the amount of time we stare at computer screens and tiny BlackBerrys, our peepers need a rest. I keep two lavender eye pillows next to my bed. The scent of lavender is calming and sleep inducing. It helps me focus on my breathing and allows my stress and anxiety to float away.

4. Relish the silence. Clanging pots, blasting TVs and radios, arguing children. There's noise everywhere in my house. When the kids have finally gone to bed and my chores are finished, I love to simply absorb the silence. Like the "quiet room" at a spa, silence can be incredibly relaxing. It helps me regroup and calm my racing mind. Occasionally, I wake up ten minutes early so I can enjoy a few minutes of solitary stretching and meditation. It's a great way to start the day. While it's tempting, don't turn on the TV or stereo . . . just enjoy the peace and quiet.

5. Get lost in a good book. When I was growing up, my school librarian always said that a good book can take you on a journey far from your everyday life. She was right. For me, an engaging novel helps transport me away from whatever is on my mind. I stop thinking about the laundry, the bills, and my next project, and instead focus on the intrigue, the characters, and what excitement will happen next in whatever I'm reading. The trick, however, is picking up a book that isn't so intriguing that you stay up all night to find out what happens!

Have Mind-Blowing Sex

Mind-blowing sex at *this* age? To some of you, it may sound like an oxymoron. But as I've learned firsthand, it *is* possible to reignite the passion in your relationship and have a satisfying sex life as you get older. True, it may not come as naturally as it did in your twenties. Hormonal changes, insecurity about how we look, stress, and lack of energy can all put the kibosh on your sex drive. But you don't have to write off sex entirely. All it means is that you may have to work a little harder to light the fires.

Back in Chapter 1, I talked about how menopausal symptoms such as vaginal dryness can throw a wrench into your sex life—and what you can do about them. But I didn't elaborate on the impact that changes in your physical appearance—and your feelings about yourself—can have on your libido. After all, if you're like me, those crow's feet and extra inches around your middle don't exactly make you feel hot and sexy. And let's face it: It isn't always easy to get aroused when you're exhausted from sleep deprivation, you're wearing an enormous maxi pad, or you've been sweating like an NBA player all day.

. . . .

"Know that you are going to die, then back up
and live each day with that truth in mind. Wake up
each morning happy to be alive."

—from *A Lotus Grows in the Mud* by Goldie Hawn

. . . .

When I'm feeling unhappy with the way I look, I find it hard to accept that anyone else finds me attractive. But the funny thing is, my husband, Billy, doesn't see what I see. He's just as attracted to me now as he was when we met fifteen years ago—maybe even more so. Go figure! Reminding myself of that fact helps me get over any feelings of self-consciousness. I also try to wear clothes that make me feel good, whether it's a favorite pair of jeans, a black T-shirt, or yoga pants. And there's nothing like a good workout to boost my confidence, so I make an extra effort to fit in my walks and weight-training sessions.

I recently met a young mother who always looks terrific. Perfect hair and makeup. I finally broke down and asked her how she does it. Her response: "I get up a half hour before my husband so I look fabulous when he gets up. I want him to leave for work excited to come home and see me." Reflecting on her thoughts, I agree. It's worth it to put effort into how you look, because it influences how you feel about yourself as well. Not only does this young mother look great, you can tell how confident she is in herself and in her relationship. Feeling good about yourself can take some work. But the result is worth it—both for you and your significant other.

Recently, I was chatting with a friend of mine at the *Today* show. We were both complaining about how hard it can be to make time for our significant others. The kids, the job, housekeeping, errands, exercise— the list can go on and on and on. And unfortunately, what usually falls to the bottom of the list is romance. I can go longer than Billy without a romantic rendezvous, but as he gently reminds me, our marriage needs attention, too.

Of course, some of you may not care about your sex life, which is totally understandable. But if it matters to the person lying next to you in bed at night, you'll need to address the issue. Otherwise, it can become a real sore spot in your relationship. I know from experience. In fact, it's the only ongoing source of tension that I have in my marriage.

My *Today* show friend was planning a weekend in Paris for himself and his wife. While he gets points for romance, such a long trip seems, well, like overkill. My suggestion, instead, is to keep it simple. Instead of saving it up for one big romantic weekend, try to light the romantic fires on a regular basis. Everyone is different. For some, sexy lingerie works. For others, it's a back rub on the couch. Or maybe it's as basic as spending some quality one-on-one time together without the kids nearby.

What I've learned over the years is that I need to feel in control of my life. Nothing is worse for my libido than feeling like I'm living in a state of chaos. If I'm on top of my work commitments and the house is basically in order, I can relax a little. I can stop worrying about the little things (Are the dishes done? Are lunches made for school? Did I get to the dry cleaner? Did I get the edits back to my publisher?) and concentrate on my husband.

Your sex life doesn't have to be on the top of your priority list every day—but if it keeps taking a backseat to other activities, both you and your partner are bound to suffer. Your significant other may feel slighted and hurt. And you'll feel guilty, which only adds more emotions to an already emotional time. So shake up your mental list of "to do" items each day . . . it isn't easy, but it does work. You don't have to get X, Y, and Z finished before you have sex. Try having sex first, then tackling X and Z, leaving Y for tomorrow.

In recent years, Billy and I have devised a few solutions to our romantic challenges. For instance, household chores and errands that, typically, we might do alone, we try to do together. This year, he came with me to our storage unit to put away our boxes of holiday decorations, just so we could spend some time together. One thing led to another, he shut the door, and we had an afternoon fling in our storage unit! We both felt great (and devious) afterward. Sometimes it just takes a few uninterrupted minutes together, and you're back on track again.

Another solution was our monthly "afternoon delight." We set up a time to meet for an afternoon of alone time at a cheap motel along the Pacific Coast Highway. For three lovely months, we rekindled our romance without interruption. We were away from home, so we couldn't be distracted by piles of work, chores, or the boys. But then the motel decided to renovate and tripled the room rate. Sadly, our hideaway is now out of our price range. But I haven't forgotten the idea! And we're eager to come up with a new alternative.

What also helps for me is making a schedule for sex. As unromantic as it sounds, I put a very discreet little red heart on my calendar for the evenings (or days) designated for "Billy and Kathy Romance." This doesn't mean I'm not up for a little spontaneity, but if I know sex is on the agenda, I can look forward to it all day and get in the mood. I can put on something sexy and maybe a little perfume. I can also avoid scheduling ten thousand other things so that I'm not thinking of, well, those ten thousand other things. This way I have a one-track mind for satisfying my husband and myself. And let's not forget that there's nothing like a little anticipation to get the motors revving!

Adding a little creativity to the mix doesn't hurt, either. We're not old dogs yet, so we can always learn new tricks, right? Sexy movies work for some, though they're not my thing. Some of my friends are considering a "passion party" (www.passionparties.com) instead, and I think it's a great idea. A sex consultant comes to your house with a variety of sensual products such as vibrators, edible creams, candles, and lingerie. You can look at everything and try on outfits you might otherwise pass by, as well as talk about, learn about, and buy products to spice up your bedroom life right in the comfort of your own home.

If shopping with your friends for, um, "personal items" seems a little too revealing, you can always head to a local adult store or shop the Web for some new toys. The Pleasure Chest, the famous sex shop in Hollywood, has shelves filled with books, videos, and other paraphernalia. Many women are opening similar female-friendly shops across the country and are offering classes, workshops, and seminars to help women improve their romantic relationships. You can also try Early to Bed in Chicago (www.early2bed.com) and Eve's Garden (www.evesgarden.com) for some private browsing.

The bottom line, though, is that mind-blowing sex doesn't have to be about crazy products or positions that you'll only see on the pay-per-view channels. It can be about showing your lover that you're interested in finding new ways to please each other. The first ingredient is feeling confident in yourself and your relationship. Why not initiate sex tonight, instead of waiting to be asked? The second ingredient is a dash of the unexpected . . . whatever that means to you. It could be silky sheets, a lacy negligee, or role playing. The third is making it a reality by finding the time for a little romance.

Of course, no matter how hard you try, the thought of sex may rank right up there with the dentist on the enjoyability scale, especially if you're experiencing vaginal dryness as the result of hormonal changes. If simple solutions such as over-the-counter lubricants and vaginal moisturizers don't seem to help, check with your physician. Other prescription options, including vaginal estrogen creams and the estrogen ring, may work for you. But remember, you won't know unless you ask.

And let's remember—sex isn't just intercourse. It's romance. It's togetherness. It's love. It's the connection, caring, and compassion that makes you feel in sync with one another. So think of other ways to flame the romantic fires. His favorite home-cooked meal by candlelight. An intensive, deep, long massage, with lots of aromatherapy oils. Spending

Find the Silver Lining

Whether you have a good or bad experience with menopause may depend on the attitude you have when entering it. Here's what the perpetually inspiring Oprah Winfrey had to say about it:

> I never expected to change the way I think about menopause; it should not be something we as women dread. I'm actually now kind of looking forward to it. Why? Because it's a chance to get better. Hot flashes—don't have to have them. Insomnia doesn't have to happen. You don't have to have all that physical stuff going on that makes you crazy. It's a chance to get better. It's your body saying to you, "Wake up!" We are going into the second act, girl! You know what I say about menopause after this show? Bring it on!

Whenever you're feeling down, follow Oprah's lead and think about all the fabulous things about moving forward with your life. Like it or not, we can't go back, so let's keep looking ahead. I like to think of it as an opportunity to feel great, get stronger, and look better—inside and out. The opportunities are endless and different for every one of us.

time together doing something you both love. And despite what a certain president said, oral sex is still sex. Surprise your partner with an unexpected dalliance. There's also the power of touch—use it to satisfy your mate the way you might have done years ago. It will bring you closer together.

Part of being closer together includes communicating. Instead of shutting out your partner, explain how you're feeling, both emotionally and physically, during this challenging time. Don't let him think you aren't attracted to him, or just keep saying "No" in hopes that he'll give up eventually. Instead, tell him what's happening—"Having sex hurts right now," "I'm exhausted and drained," or "It's hard for me to be romantic when I feel so uncomfortable." Failure to communicate can breed resentment and hurt feelings. Being open and honest, on the other hand, creates a different kind of intimacy. It can really generate compassion and understanding, and deepen your friendship.

Stay Young at Heart

Sometimes it's hard for me to believe that my life could be half over. But then again, so much has happened to me in the past forty-four years. I've grown up, graduated from high school, gone to college, started a business, fallen in love, fallen in love again, gotten married, had babies, and watched them grow before my very eyes. When I think about all that has transpired, I realize how much time (weeks, months, years, decades) I have left to experience more laughs, tears, talks, walks, hugs, kisses, and smiles—as well as new adventures.

When it comes to living life, I think it's important to remember that age is just a number. Just because we're in our forties, fifties, or sixties, it doesn't mean that we can't go back to school, run a marathon, or wear designer jeans. In fact, there's never been a better time to strive for new goals and add some excitement to your life. Whether you want to switch careers, start a business, write a book, travel the world, or train for a triathalon, you now have the wisdom and experience to succeed.

In other words, reinvent yourself! Ask yourself, "Am I the woman that I want to be? Is this the life that I want to lead? Is there something that I've been aching to do that I haven't done yet?" Life isn't over after menopause. Now may be the perfect opportunity to pursue your passions, take on new challenges, or simply do what you've been wanting to do for years (finish every Jane Austen novel, learn to play tennis, do volunteer work, or rent a villa in Italy).

. . . .

"Menopause has forced me to be courageous. Life isn't just coming to me anymore, like it did when I was younger. Now I have to make choices and go out and get what I want. In that way, it's challenging. But I'm also finding that I'm up for it. For example, I've had a fantasy all of my life about owning horses. I'm terrified of doing it. But my husband and I have already started transforming our property into an equestrian center. I figure why keep putting it off? What am I waiting for? Why not *now*?"

—Molly, age fifty-three

. . . .

Keep a notebook in your purse. Whenever a new idea pops into your mind, write it down. It can be something as silly as learning to skateboard or as serious as running for a local political office. Research each idea and focus on the one or two you're really interested in achieving. Remind yourself that you can do anything you set your mind to. Don't let your age dictate what you can do; just get out there and do it. If you decide it isn't for you, no problem—try something else. Don't forget, you're only as old as you act!

Turning the Page

As you enter this new chapter in your life, I want you to embark on a new journey filled with excitement, energy, love, laughter, and self-fulfillment. Don't let your changing body keep you from feeling good about yourself and making the most of your life. There's no need to pause for menopause. You're the writer of this next great adventure. It's up to you to make it a page-turner!

Appendix

Kathy's Favorites!

Exercise

Podfitness.com: Download my workouts from this Web site, and I can be your real personal trainer on your iPod or MP3 player. Whatever your goal, I'll coach your every step.

KathyKaehlerfitness.com: Come find out what I'm up to! On this site, you can read all about my Health-E-tips, or buy my latest books and videos online. You can also send me an e-mail with any of your fitness questions.

Fitness Gear

Enell Sports Bra: This ultrasupportive sports bra, with a hook-and-eye closure, is specially designed for large-breasted women. When I introduced Drew Barrymore to it, she exclaimed, "This bra is going to change my life!" To purchase one or find a local retailer, visit www.enell.com.

X2 Vest: If you watch the *Today* show, you may have seen me wearing this weighted vest on a segment with Katie Couric. It can boost the intensity of your walking workouts so you burn even more calories. For details, go to www.x2vest.com.

Gymp3.com: Visit this site for my audio fitness program.

Nikewomen.com: I love my Nikes because they fit so well and perform for me every time. You'll never see me in another pair of workout shoes!

Spriproducts.com: This online retailer sells just about every fitness product under the sun. You can find most of the equipment needed for my workouts right here.

Super Rope: If you know me, you know that I love to jump rope. The Super Rope is the only kind of rope that I'll use. 414-771-0849.

Food/Nutrition

The Dish on Eating Healthy and Being Fabulous!: Co-written by my friend Carolyn O'Neil, RD, this fun, informative, and practical book explains how to eat healthy, whether you're at home, dining out, traveling, or entertaining. It also offers insightful tips and recipes from well-known chefs, restaurateurs, and other experts. Go to www.carolynoneil.com.

Dr. Praeger's Sensible Foods: Developed by two cardiac surgeons, these yummy frozen foods are low in cholesterol and saturated fats, and are free of preservatives and artificial ingredients. I'm a big fan of the broccoli patties and veggie burgers. To find a retail outlet near you, go to www.drpraegers.com.

Givemepopcorn.com: This Web site has all sorts of gourmet popcorn products. I especially love the Baby White Gourmet Popcorn, which is hull-less—so it doesn't get stuck in your teeth.

Health by Chocolate: I discovered these antioxidant-packed dark chocolate bars at Whole Foods. They were formulated by a dermatologist specifically for women, and are enhanced with nutrients such as calcium, vitamin D, soy, and lycopene. To learn more, go to www.healthbychocolate.com.

Kagome 100% Juices: I love these fruit and vegetable juices! They're completely natural, with no added sugar, artificial flavors, or preservatives. To find a retail outlet, go to www.kagome.us.

PopcornPopper.com: Here's where you can get my beloved Whirley Pop Popcorn Popper, along with other fun popcorn products.

Propel Fitness Water: I don't know about you, but I get tired of drinking plain water. This lightly flavored water is infused with vitamins and minerals, and has only 10 calories per eight-ounce serving. For details, go to www.propelwater.com.

Sexuality

Early2bed.com: This is a fun site to visit with your best friend or your partner. Order something that you never thought you would use. You may be surprised!

Evesgarden.com: Here's another go-to place for adult toys, DVDs and videos, massage oils, and the like.

Passion Parties: Learn how to host your own passion party, or browse around in the Passion Boutique. Go to www.passionparties.com.

Skin Care

Total Block: I never leave home without a bottle of this sunblock. I use both the clear and tinted formulas. It isn't greasy, and it blocks both UVA and UVB rays. For more info, go to www.totalblock.com.

Nerida Joy Skincare: I started getting facials from Nerida Joy about fifteen years ago. Her client list includes celebrity A-listers such as Courteney Cox and Jennifer Garner. To purchase her products or learn about common skin woes such as hyperpigmentation and rosacea, visit www.neridajoyskincare.com.

Women's Health

Bonehealthequation.com: Everything you ever wanted to know about strengthening your bones.

DrDonnica.com: This Web site, founded by Donnica L. Moore, MD, a leading women's health expert and advocate, has information on topics including breast health, menopause, and weight control.

Index